Treat Your Own
Knee Arthritis

by
Jim Johnson, PT

This book was designed to provide accurate information in regard to the subject matter covered. It is sold with the understanding that the author is not engaged in rendering medical, psychological, or other professional services. If expert assistance is required, the services of a professional should be sought.

Anatomical Drawings by Eunice Johnson
Exercise Drawings by Amberly Powell
Copyright © 2011 Jim Johnson
All Rights Reserved

This edition published by
Dog Ear Publishing
4010 W. 86th Street, Ste H
Indianapolis, IN 46268

www.dogearpublishing.net

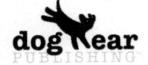

ISBN: 978-1-4575-4017-2
Library of Congress Control Number: Applied For
This book is printed on acid-free paper.

Printed in the United States of America

How This Book Is Set Up

✓ Gain a new perspective of knee arthritis in *Chapter 1*.

✓ Be aware of the typical course that knee arthritis takes in *Chapter 2*.

✓ Learn how you can treat knee arthritis yourself in *Chapters 3 through 7*.

✓ Monitor your progress with the tools in *Chapter 8*.

Why Is The Print In This Book So Big?

People who read my books sometimes wonder why the print is so big in many of them. Some tend to think it's because I'm trying to make a little book bigger or a short book longer.

Actually, the main reason I use bigger print is for the same reason I intentionally write short books, usually under 100 pages–it's just plain easier to read and get the information quicker!

You see, the books I write address common, everyday problems that people of *all* ages have. In other words, the "typical" reader of my books could be a teenager, a busy housewife, a CEO, a construction worker, or a retired senior citizen with poor eyesight. Therefore, by writing books with larger print that are short and to the point, *everyone* can get the information quickly and with ease. After all, what good is a book full of useful information if nobody ever finishes it?

Contents

I have given my best effort to ensure that this book is entirely based upon scientific evidence and not on intuition, single case reports, opinions of authorities, anecdotal evidence, or unsystematic clinical observations. Where I do state my opinion in this book, it is directly stated as such.

—Jim Johnson, P.T.

Here's What's Going On In Your Knee

Knee arthritis is one of the most common conditions I treat as a physical therapist. Unfortunately, it's also one of the *least* understood conditions people have. For example, if a doctor tells a patient that they have knee arthritis, many might think it's just because of old age–which is actually a really *bad* way to think about knee arthritis.

While it *is* true that getting older definitely makes one more susceptible to getting knee arthritis, *aging alone does not cause it.* We know this because not all older adults will develop knee arthritis. For instance…

- researchers studied 463 subjects (Miller 2001)
- they were all 65 years or older
- all had knee pain on most days of the week
- X-rays were taken of their knees
- only 52% of subjects had knee arthritis

So out of 463 people, all of whom were at least 65 years old, only about *half* had knee arthritis. Apparently knee arthritis and getting older don't necessarily *have* to go hand-in-hand.

Yet others with knee arthritis are under the impression that their knees have simply, well, worn out over time. If this were true, and our knees will only last so long before hopelessly breaking down, then studies should show us that people who use their knees the most have the most arthritis, right? Well, let's take a quick look. Here's some research that has been done on individuals who probably push their knees harder than most on a weekly basis, *runners…*

- 45 long-distance runners were followed for an average of 12 years (Chakravarty 2008)

- researchers also followed a control group of 53 individuals who were matched to the runners for age, education level, and occupation

- everyone was over 50 years of age and had x-rays taken of their knees at the beginning and end of the study

- runners ran an average of three and a half hours a week, while the control group ran an average of a half hour a week

- after 12 years, runners did not have any more knee arthritis than the control group

So if the weekly pounding of long-distance running really does wear out your knees, one would think that knees subjected to over 3 hours a week of running would show *more* wear and tear than knees subjected to only 30 minutes a week– but that wasn't the case. Everybody's knees in the study showed similar degrees of arthritis at the end of the 12-year follow-up.

This is a pretty typical finding too in the research on running and knee arthritis…

- one study using x-rays followed a group of 50+ year old runners and non-runners for nine years (Lane 1998). Runners ran an average of 25 miles a week. *9-year x-ray results showed that knee arthritis progressed to the same degree in both groups.*

- another study, also using x-rays, followed runners and non-runners for eight years (Panush 1995). These runners ran an average of 28 miles a week. *8-year follow-up showed no notable differences in knee x-rays between the two groups.*

Obviously getting knee arthritis isn't as simple as using your knees a lot and wearing them out. Every time the foot hits the ground during running, the compressive forces at the knee joint have been shown to be about 10 times your body weight (Messier 2008). Applying this fact to a 150-pound runner, who has an average of 400 foot strikes per foot per mile, *each knee* endures about 300 tons of force *every* mile. However despite this kind of beating, the studies clearly point out that people who regularly use their knees in this manner have no more knee arthritis than anyone else.

In the pages to come, you'll see that your knees are *not* like automobile tires that only have so much life left in them before they wear out. While most readers already know that knee arthritis involves the loss of knee cartilage, research is now showing us there's a lot more to it than that. The fact of the matter is that knee arthritis is actually a condition that involves the *entire* knee, with the knee suffering from some *very specific* problems. And it's the purpose of this book to show you which of these problems you can treat, on your own, that will get your knee working and feeling a whole lot better. Having said that, let's get a little more familiar with some of the key structures that can be affected in knee arthritis.

The Parts of Your Knee You *Need* to Know About

Before you can start treating your own knee arthritis, you've got to know what you're dealing with. After all, what mechanic would try to fix a car engine he knew absolutely nothing about? Of course a few readers have probably had that experience before…

Now instead of just listing all the parts of your knee, and then giving you a boring medical definition, we're going to go over the knee's structures by taking a look at pictures of it from the *inside* out. Up first is the basic framework of your knee, *the bones…*

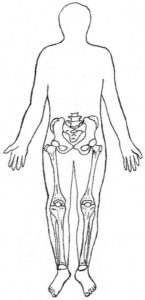

Figure 1. The bones of the upper and lower leg that come together to form your knees.

A look at Figure 1 quickly tells us that the knee is made up of more than just one bone. The following pictures give us a closer look, and reveal to us that the knee is actually made up of three distinct bones; the *femur* (upper leg bone), the *tibia* (the lower leg bone) and the *patella* (your kneecap).

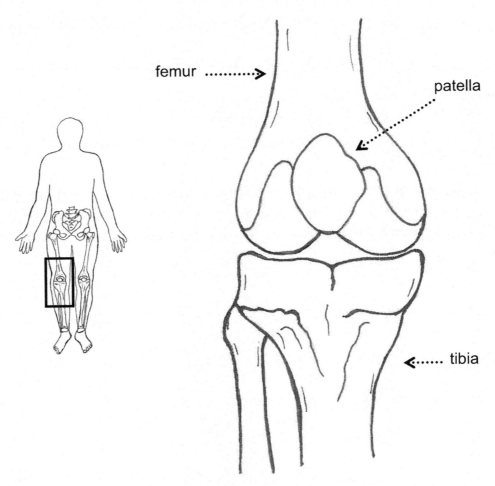

Figure 2. Front view of the three bones that make up the right knee joint.

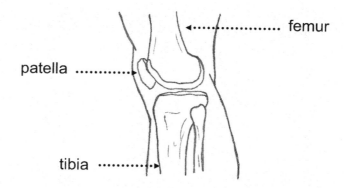

Figure 3. Side view of the three
bones that make up the knee joint.

the articular cartilage

Now that you have an idea of what bones make up your knee, it's important to note that where they do come together and meet, their ends are coated with a substance called *articular cartilage*. Being very slick and smooth, it's a big job of the articular cartilage to decrease friction between the bones and help them move smoothly upon one another. Here's a side view showing where the articular cartilage coats the ends of your knee bones…

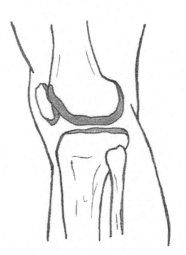

Figure 4. Shaded areas show where the knee bones are
coated with smooth articular cartilage.

Here are a few more pictures at different angles. This one is good because it shows the cartilage that is located on the *back* of your knee cap. Yep, you've got cartilage there too!

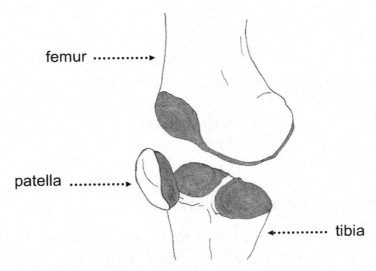

Figure 5. Shaded areas show where the articular cartilage is.

And this one shows the areas of cartilage with the knee cap removed and the knee in a *bent* position.

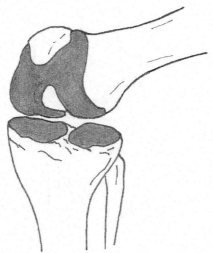

Figure 6. Shaded areas show where the articular cartilage is.

Know that normal articular cartilage is a white, smooth, firm substance that is made up of cells called *chondrocytes*. However unlike other tissues in your body, like the skin or muscles, articular cartilage has *no* blood supply going to it. In other words, there are no small blood vessels going directly to it to provide life sustaining nutrients. So just how do these tiny little chondrocytes get their nutrition?

To answer that question, we have to take a microscopic look at how the articular cartilage is made up. If you take a piece of articular cartilage from your knee joint, and look at it from the *side* under a powerful microscope, you'd see that it actually has several different layers to it. Check out this picture and you'll see what I mean…

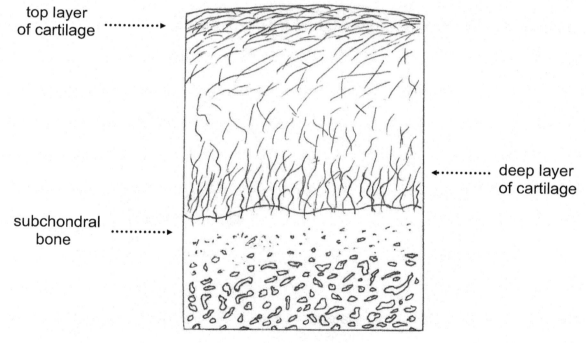

Figure 7. A sideview of the different layers of the articular cartilage in the knee. Note how the knee cartilage eventually blends with the underlying bone.

As you can easily see, there are several different layers to the articular cartilage. Scientists believe that the top layer gets its nutrition from a liquid floating around in the knee joint known as *synovial fluid* (more on that stuff in a few pages).

And the deeper layer of cartilage? It's most likely that it gets its nutrition from the *subchondral bone* it's right next to. In case you're confused, the subchondral bone is just a fancy name for the bone that sits *right under* the layers of cartilage.

the meniscus

Now even though the ends of the tibia and femur are coated with this super-slick articular cartilage stuff that help them move smoothly upon each another, you can see looking back at Figure 6, that the ends of the two bones are shaped *very* differently from each other–not exactly what you'd call "a perfect fit."

So, in order to help this situation, there are two little structures *in between* the two bones called the *medial meniscus*, and *the lateral meniscus*. Pronounced mun-iss-cuss , here's what they look like sitting in your knee…

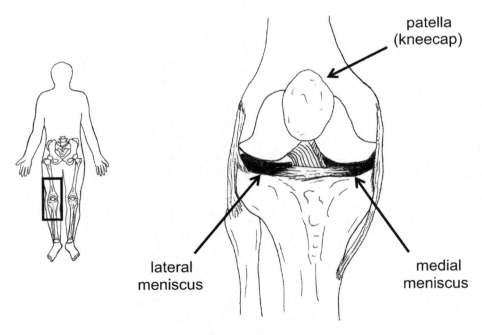

Figure 8. Front view of the medial and lateral meniscus of the right knee.

Since the upper bone of the knee, the femur, has two *round* parts that sit directly on the *flatter* tibia bone, you can see how the medial and lateral meniscus really help improve the fit between the two bones.

Now that you've seen what the medial and lateral meniscus look like from the front, let's lift up the femur a bit to get a better look at things...

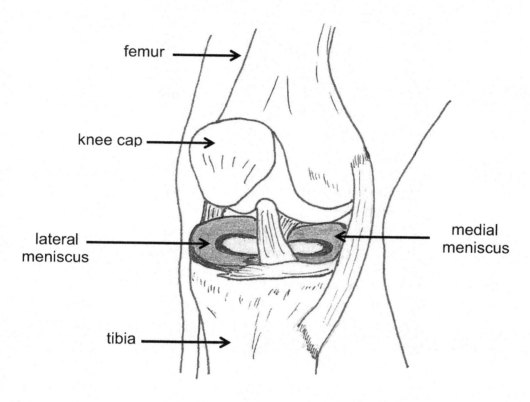

Figure 9. How the medial and lateral meniscus sit in the right knee joint.

Like the articular cartilage that coats the end of the bones, the medial and lateral meniscus are also made of cartilage, however it's a different kind called *fibrocartilage*.

Besides helping the femur and tibia fit together a little better, the medial and lateral meniscus also help out with shock absorption and work hard to transmit forces across the knee more efficiently. This last picture reveals how different the medial and lateral meniscus really are in shape…

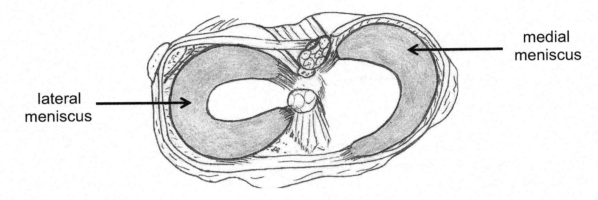

medial
meniscus

lateral
meniscus

Figure 10. Overhead view of the medial and lateral meniscus.

the ligaments

Okay. Up to this point we've got two bones covered with smooth articular cartilage on their ends, that are neatly fitted together with two pieces of fibrocartilage in between them. So the next question is, what *keeps* them together? Well, it's a specialized connective tissue known as a *ligament*.

While there are many different ligaments in and around the knee, some big, some small, we're going to take a look at the major ones. There are four of them, and they are:

- the anterior cruciate ligament
- the posterior cruciate ligament
- the medial collateral ligament
- the lateral collateral ligament

Since it's the job of the ligaments to hold the bones together, it's logical that they'd have to run from one bone to another. Let's see exactly where they are in the knee…

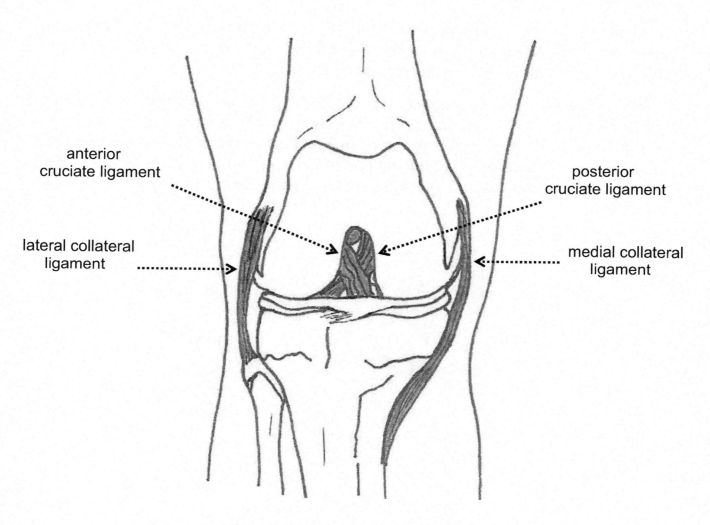

anterior
cruciate ligament

posterior
cruciate ligament

lateral collateral
ligament

medial collateral
ligament

Figure 11. Front view of the four major ligaments of the right knee that help hold the bones in place.

Did you notice that the two ligaments in the middle cross each other and make an "x"? That's why they were named the *cruciate* ligaments, because "cruciate" comes from the Latin word "crux" –which means cross. By the way, if you've ever heard of an athlete tearing their "ACL", it was the **A**nterior **C**ruciate **L**igament that they tore. Ouch!

While these four ligaments work hard all day to help hold your knee bones in place, don't think that they just sit there stiff as a board. If that was the case, you wouldn't be able to move your knee around very much!

So just how do these ligaments work? Well, a ligament will allow a certain amount of motion to take place in the knee, but, if a bone starts going *too far* in one direction, growing tension in the ligament stops it. By working this way, the ligaments can both *permit* a certain amount of knee motion, as well as *limit* it. Take a look at these examples and you'll see how the ligaments react as you move your knee around…

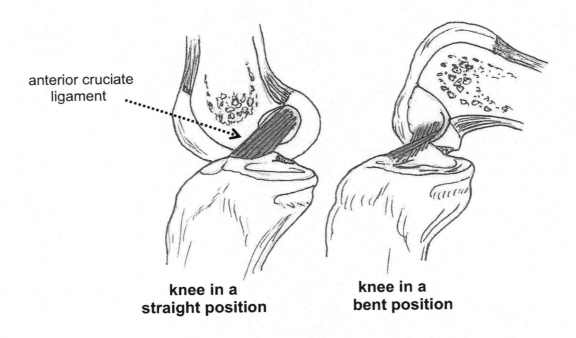

anterior cruciate
ligament

**knee in a
straight position**

**knee in a
bent position**

Figure 12. A side view showing how the anterior cruciate ligament reacts when you bend and straighten your knee.

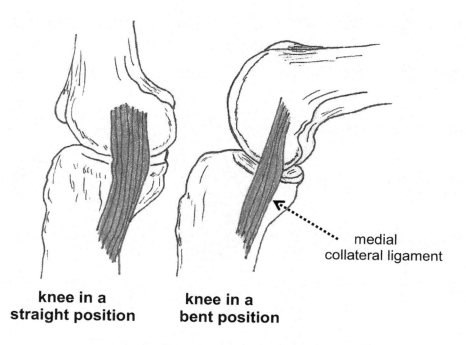

**knee in a
straight position**   **knee in a
bent position**

Figure 13. A side view showing how the
medial collateral ligament reacts when you
bend and straighten your knee.

the synovial membrane

I doubt a lot of readers have heard of this knee structure. The *synovial membrane* is like a "sleeve" that fits neatly around your knee joint and envelopes it. This is what it looks like :

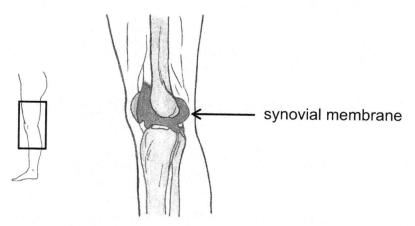

Figure 14. The synovial membrane

Interesting structure, isn't it? Think of the synovial membrane kind of like a plastic wrap that clings closely to the entire knee joint. Here are a few more pictures to give you a better look…

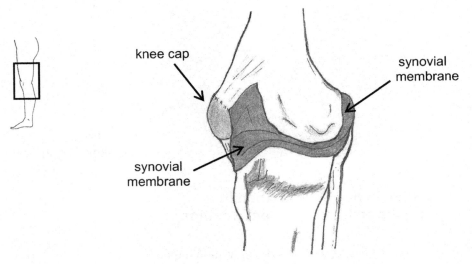

Figure 15. A side view of the synovial membrane

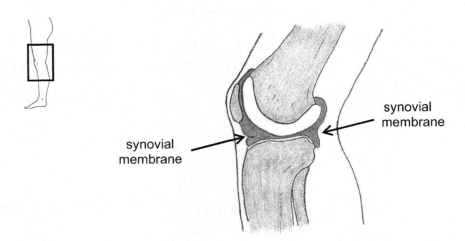

Figure 16. A cut-out side view of the synovial membrane. Note how the synovium wraps itself around the two bones and "seals in" the knee joint.

So what does the synovial membrane do? Well, it lines the joint and makes that substance we talked about on page 8 called *synovial fluid*. Synovial fluid is a must-have to your knee, because it floats around and provides nutrients to the cartilage in your knee. Additionally, it also helps lubricate your knee joint.

the bursae

Have you ever heard of bursitis? A lot of people have. It's common in the shoulder, and you get it when you have a problem with a small structure called a *bursae* (pronounced burr-sah). So what's a bursae?

Well, bursae in general are flat, sac-like structures that are located *all* throughout your body. If you've ever seen a deflated whoopie cushion, well, that's about what they look like. It's the main job of these bursae to reduce friction and make things slide a whole lot easier, particularly in areas where structures have a tendency to rub together a lot–like where a tendon passes right over a bone.

Now normally these little guys contain a small amount of fluid, however if they get really irritated for any number of reason, well, they can really swell up and cause you a lot of pain–and then you've got bursitis. You've got a bunch of bursae around your knee joint, and here's a picture of some of the major ones…

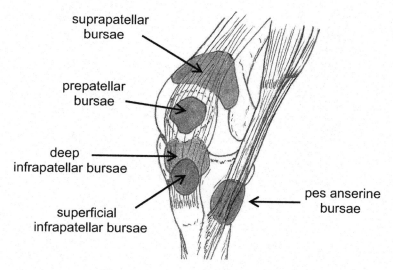

Figure 17. Some of the major bursae around the right knee.

the muscles

We're finally to the last and outermost structure of your knee, the muscles which make your knee move. While there are quite a few of them in and around the knee, I just want you to be familiar with two major groups in particular–the *quadriceps* and the *hamstrings*. As the following pictures show, the quadriceps muscles take up most of the *front* of your thigh, while the hamstrings make up most of the *back*. Here's a look at where they are…

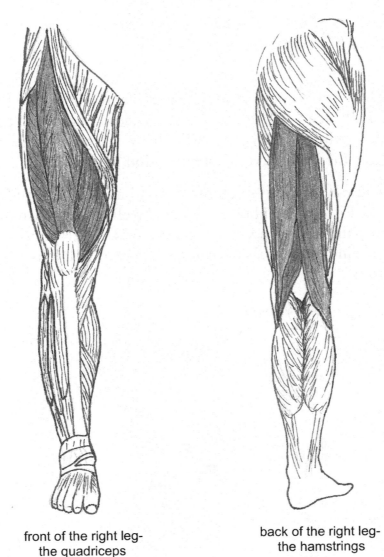

front of the right leg-
the quadriceps

back of the right leg-
the hamstrings

Figure 18. Shaded areas showing the quadriceps and hamstring muscle groups.

What Happens to Your Knee When You Get Arthritis

Now that you're a little more familiar with the parts of your knee, we can talk about some of the changes that can take place when you have arthritis.

Probably the first change that comes to mind is that of the cartilage. While it is true that arthritic knees show a loss of cartilage, *arthritis is really a disorder of the whole joint.* Having said that, here's a list of some of the changes that are commonly found in the knees of people with arthritis:

- loss of the *articular cartilage* that coats the ends of the bones

- changes in the *subchondral bone* (the bone under the cartilage). Frequently seen on MRI scans are abnormal areas in the bone called bone marrow lesions, or BML's.

- small outgrowths of bone called *osteophytes* (bone spurs) can form at the edges of the bones

- the *synovial membrane* often becomes thicker and can become inflamed

- tears in the *meniscus* are also a common finding

As you can see, there's a lot more going on in the arthritic knee than just the loss of cartilage. With all these changes taking place, one begins to wonder, where exactly does the pain come from?

What Causes The Pain When You Get Arthritis

For a knee structure to cause you pain, it has to have nerve pain fibers going to it, simply because it's the nerves that are responsible for carrying pain signals up to your brain telling you that you're hurting. Therefore, anything in your knee that has nerve pain fibers going to it *could* be a source of knee pain–and that's where the guessing game begins.

The problem here is that there are *a lot* of structures in your knee that contain pain fibers, such as the synovial membrane, the meniscus, and the bone to name a few–so good luck figuring out exactly which one(s) in particular are the exact culprit. About the only knee structure we can safely *rule out* is the articular cartilage that can be seen disappearing on x-rays–knee cartilage actually has *no* pain fibers going to it, and therefore cannot produce any pain. Isn't that something–the number one structure people associate with knee arthritis can't even give you pain!

So what else have we got? Well, another way of trying to figure out what's causing the pain in knee arthritis is to pinpoint the knee structures that are abnormal, and then blame them. However, there's a problem with this approach too–you can find many knee abnormalities in people that have *no pain*. For instance…

- researchers studied 319 subjects that had knee arthritis on x-ray. *Only 47% of them had any knee pain* (Hannan 2000).

- another study looked at 50 people that had knee arthritis but had no pain. *30% of them had BML's, or bone marrow lesions on MRI* (Felson 2001).

- In this study, 154 patients over 45 years of age with knee arthritis, were compared to 49 subjects over 45 years of age that had no knee pain or knee arthritis (Bhattacharyya 2003). MRI scans found meniscus tears in 91% of arthritic knees. However, *76% of those people with pain-free knees also had meniscus tears.*

From these studies, you can quickly see the problem with trying to figure out the source of one's pain by looking for abnormalities in the knee. As these studies show us, there's a lot of people walking around with *no* knee pain that have knee arthritis and meniscus tears. While that might seem unbelievable, it's true and well documented in the published arthritis research.

So now what? How does one go about figuring out what's causing their arthritic knee pain?

Well, with the current technology, the most realistic answer is it's just not possible to precisely pinpoint what structure(s) are causing the pain in many cases. However, before you get *too* discouraged, let me also add that you don't necessarily *have* to know the exact source of your knee pain to get rid of it…

Perhaps a Better Approach to Getting Rid of Knee Pain

So far in this chapter we've been looking at knee arthritis from a *structural* point of view. We know from x-rays and MRI's that cartilage wears down, the underlying bone changes, the meniscus can tear, and so on. We've also noted from the research studies, that in many cases, you can have these changes in your knee and still be pain-free–which leaves us a little empty-handed at times trying to explain what exactly causes arthritis pain.

However dig into the research on arthritic knee *function*, and you'll get a little different perspective on things. By function, I'm talking about how your knee works and performs. For example, how strong are your knee muscles? How well can you bend or straighten your knee?

So what does the research on arthritic knee function show us? A lot. Here's an example…

- researchers went out into the community and randomly selected 462 men and women that were over 65 years of age (Slemenda 1997)

- x-rays were taken of their knees, as well as the strength of the subject's quadriceps muscles, an important stabilizer of the knee

- it was found that men and women with knee arthritis had much weaker quadriceps muscles than those with *no* knee arthritis

- researchers also noted that women with *painful* knee arthritis had much weaker quadriceps muscles than those with *non-painful* knee arthritis

It's interesting that the people with knee arthritis had much weaker leg muscles than the people without knee arthritis. Even more interesting, is that among the women *with* arthritis, those with pain had more weakness than those without pain.

Hmm. Apparently there are *other* problems going on in the arthritic knee other than just the structural abnormalities we see pictured all so clearly on X-rays and MRI's. In the above study, the researchers could actually predict who had knee arthritis and who had *painful* knee arthritis–simply by looking at whose leg muscles were working the best!

Okay, *now* we're getting somewhere–and we're in a lot more optimistic position. In this book, we're not going to be concerned so much with things such as cartilage loss, a torn meniscus or bone spurs. We know from *many* studies that it's *quite* possible for people to live just fine with these kinds of changes in the knee– so we're going to just let them be.

And what are we going to focus on? *Improving the functioning of your knee.* Why? Because functional problems, like improperly working knee muscles, seem much more related to one having pain, than how bad pictures of your knee look on an x-ray or MRI. Therefore, this book is going to lead you step-by-step through a series of "tune-ups" that are specifically designed to get your knee in good working order. If you've got weak knee muscles, we're going to zero in on the key ones and make them stronger. If your knee is stiff, well, we're going to loosen it up–and so on.

The plan is sound. Pain is the result of something not functioning properly–so if we improve the functioning of your knee, your symptoms will also improve. I've been using this principle with patients for over nineteen years now, and as you'll soon see, we have some pretty good studies that show it *really* works!

> ## *Quick Review*
>
> ✓ knee arthritis is not simply the loss of cartilage. In reality, the *entire* knee is affected.
>
> ✓ major structures of the knee that are affected in knee arthritis include the articular cartilage, the subchondral bone, the meniscus, and the synovial membrane. Problems with the ligaments and bursae are also common findings in knee arthritis.
>
> ✓ it is hard to pinpoint the exact cause of knee pain because many structures in the knee are capable of producing pain. Additionally, many people have structural abnormalities in their knees, but *no pain.*
>
> ✓ a better approach to treating knee arthritis, as opposed to treating structural abnormalties that may or may not be the cause of pain, is to improve the functioning of your knee.
>
> ✓ pain is the result of something not functioning properly. Improve the functioning of your knee, and the pain will improve.

 # What's Likely to Happen to Your Knee Over the Long Run

It's crossed the mind of everyone who has knee arthritis: "What's going to happen to my knee in the future?"

As a physical therapist, I have patients ask me these kinds of questions all the time. How long will my back hurt? Will my rotator cuff tear eventually heal? When will my plantar fasciitis go away? We all want to know if things will get better or worse when we have a health problem, and medicine has come up with a way to scientifically address these kinds of issues–by conducting what are known as *natural history* studies.

Simply put, a natural history study takes a group of people with a specific medical problem, and then follows them over time to see how their condition changes. As you might guess, the best natural history studies follow patients for many, many years, and the less medical interference the better–so researchers can tell what a condition does on its own, *naturally*.

So are there any natural history studies done on knee arthritis? Plenty. Over the years, I've read every one I could get my hands on, and quickly realized you can roughly divide them up into two kinds. The first mainly sets out to see how people's knee arthritis progresses *radiographically* (on x-rays) over time, and they go something like this:

- researchers get together a group of people with knee arthritis

- x-rays are taken of their knees at the beginning of the study, and again after a period of years

- at the end of the study, the two sets of x-rays, taken years apart, are compared with each other, to see how much the arthritic knees have changed over time

Sounds like a good way to figure out how arthritic knees do over the long run, huh? Well, not so fast. While natural history studies that follow changes in knee structure can certainly tell us how your knee might *look* on an x-ray in 10 years, they still don't tell us how your arthritic knee might *feel* in 10 years.

The main problem here, is that the degree of arthritis seen on x-ray pictures just don't match-up with pain levels in many cases. While you might think that people with *a little* knee arthritis, will always have less pain than people with *a lot* of knee arthritis, that's simply not what the research finds.

To begin with, recall from the study in Chapter One (Hannan 2000), that only around 50% of people with knee arthritis on an x-ray even have pain–which means the other 50% with knee arthritis have *no pain.* Think about it, studies show that there are a lot of people walking around with knee arthritis, yet have *no* pain.

Well, but maybe the people with knee arthritis and no pain just don't have *as bad* of arthritis? Makes sense, but that's not the case either. Consider this study:

- researchers studied 123 patients that were waiting to have a knee replacement (Barker 2004)
- knee x-rays were taken, and researchers assessed how much pain they were having
- interestingly, *no association was found between how much a knee hurt and the degree of knee arthritis seen on x-rays*

Apparently it's far from being an open and shut case that the worse your arthritis is, the worse your pain is going to be. Let's look at another study…

- 31 patients with knee arthritis were examined eight years apart (Massardo 1989)
- knee x-rays were taken, and researchers assessed their pain levels
- at the end of the eight-year study period, it was found that four patients had *improved* symptoms, and three of those four actually developed *more severe* arthritis on their x-rays!
- equally striking was the complete lack of association between x-ray and symptomatic changes with time

Now there's an interesting finding–some people's knees in the study began to feel *better* over the years as their arthritis got *worse!*

While the idea might seem strange that x-ray pictures of your knee can have little to do with how bad your knee feels, it's what the research has found in many studies. In fact, a research study (Bedson 2008) published in the peer-reviewed journal *BMC Musculoskeletal Disorders*, conducted an exhaustive systematic search of all the available scientific literature on the subject, and concluded that "radiographic knee osteoarthritis is an imprecise guide to the likelihood that knee pain or disability will be present." Having worked hands-on with patients for over 19 years, I couldn't have put it better myself.

Okay. So if looking at x-ray pictures of our knees can't tell us much about how they'll be doing in the long run, then what can?

Well, I mentioned a few pages ago that you can roughly divide up the natural history studies on knee arthritis into two types–which now brings us to the *second* kind that focuses more on how knee *symptoms* change over time. As you will see, these studies will help us better answer the question, "What's going to happen to my knee in the future?", simply because researchers have followed people's arthritic knees for years, and then asked subjects how they *feel*. Let's have a look at one that has a fairly long follow-up period...

- 63 subjects with knee arthritis were followed for 11 years (Spector 1992)

- at the end of the study, subjects were asked if they thought their pain was improved, the same, or worse. 56% thought their pain had gotten worse.

- subjects also rated their knee pain on a 100 point visual analogue scale, where 0 is no pain, and 100 is the worst pain

- in the beginning of the study, the average knee pain score for the whole group was 53

- 11 years later, the average knee pain score for the group was 48

- the researchers concluded that most patients with knee arthritis do not deteriorate symptomatically over an 11-year period

This study is notable because it has a pretty long follow-up period, eleven years, and it shows us that it's simply not the case that *all* arthritic knees are doomed to become more painful in the future. When patients were asked, only a little over half subjectively felt that their knee pain had gotten worse. And when patients filled out a pain scale, no increases in pain levels could be objectively measured. Let's look at one more…

- 110 patients with knee osteoarthritis were recruited from a rheumatology clinic and followed for 8 years (Dieppe 2000)

- at the beginning of the study, 5% had no pain, 35% had mild pain, 35% had moderate pain, and 25% had severe pain

- after 8 years, 3% had no pain, 25% had mild pain, 45% had moderate pain, and 27% had severe pain

- after 8 years, patients were also asked how much they thought the condition of their knee had changed. Interestingly, 20% thought their knee had gotten better overall and 17% thought it was the same.

Here again, we see that it's far from being a given that the pain from knee arthritis only continues to get worse over time. In fact, 20% of the patients followed in this study actually felt that their knee arthritis had gotten *better* overall during the 8-year study period.

So what are we to make of all these studies? What do their findings mean for the person with knee arthritis that is wondering what's likely to happen to their knee over the long run?

Well, for one, the natural history studies give us a little better view of what *really* happens to arthritic knees, so forget what your friend at work or grandma told you. Scientific studies that have followed huge groups of people for many years tell us it's a big mistake to look down at your knee and only expect the pain to get worse as time goes on. As they've clearly shown us, there are many people whose knee pain remains quite stable over the years, and in a significant amount, the pain actually gets *better*.

On the other hand though, they do also make us aware of the fact that a certain percentage of knees *will* go on to feel worse. But before this fact gets you too discouraged, I also need to point out that there are many studies that have been done on people who have reached the "worse" category, and through simple treatments, have managed to successfully move into the "improved" category.

Which treatments work the best? Well, the studies we've just gone over don't really give us many specific answers in that department–however there are plenty of other studies that do. And that's exactly what the remainder of this book is all about: the best treatments that will improve knee functioning and decrease knee pain in the shortest amount of time–*that you can do all on your own.*

Quick Review

✓ there are natural history studies that have followed arthritis patients for many years to see what happens to their knees over time

✓ in many cases, the degree of arthritis seen on x-rays doesn't match up with pain levels. Research studies have shown that some knees with a little arthritis can hurt a lot, and some knees with a lot of arthritis don't hurt at all.

✓ natural history studies that follow knee arthritis patients for many years to see how pain levels change have revealed that the course of knee arthritis is variable from person to person

✓ many arthritic knees do not become more painful over time, and in fact, a significant number actually show *improved* symptoms over time

✓ while some arthritic knees do continue to feel worse over time, many studies have shown that there are simple treatments that can significantly improve knee pain and functioning

Tune-Up #1: How to Make Your Knee *Much* Stronger

The first thing we're going to tune-up is your *knee muscles*. But why? What makes us think there could be anything wrong with them?

Well, as we touched on at the end of Chapter 1, researchers that have tested the muscles of people with knee arthritis have come across some *pretty* interesting findings…

- 77 patients with symptomatic knee arthritis were compared to 63 people that had *no* knee pain (Hassan 2001)

- all subjects had the strength of their quadriceps muscles tested

- results showed that the people with painful arthritis had much weaker quadriceps muscles than the people with no knee pain

---

and

- 90 subjects with knee arthritis, 45 men and 45 women, were compared to 104 control subjects without knee pain (Fisher 1997)

- all subjects had the strength of their quadriceps muscles tested

- it was found that the subjects with knee arthritis had much weaker quadriceps muscles than the subjects with no knee pain

---

These two studies give us some strong clues that people with knee arthritis have leg muscles that simply aren't as strong as they should be–and other studies comparing arthritic knees to normal knees have found the exact same thing…

> - this study looked at 10 people that had arthritis in just _one_ of their knees (Hurley 1993)
>
> - the strength of their quadriceps muscle was tested in _both_ knees
>
> - it was found that the quadriceps muscle in the arthritic knee was actually 40% _weaker_ than their other normal, non-arthritic knee

As you've probably gathered by now, the muscle that stands out as being the weakest in particular is the _quadriceps_ muscle. If you don't remember what it looks like, here's another look at this problem muscle…

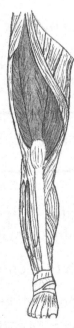

Figure 19. Shaded area shows the quadriceps muscle which has been shown to be weak in people with knee arthritis.

As you can see, it's a pretty big muscle that takes up most of your upper thigh. So what's it do? Well, if you happen to be sitting in a chair, go ahead and kick your leg out. This motion is actually one of the main jobs of the quadriceps muscle–it straightens your leg out.

Now try this. Stand up from a sitting position, and as you're doing this, put one hand on the front of your thigh. Did you feel the quadriceps muscle under your hand get harder and tighten as you began to rise? This is yet another important function of this muscle. When your foot is planted firmly on the floor, the quadriceps works hard to pull you up into a standing position.

Along with these kinds of activities, the quadriceps muscle is also largely responsible for you being able to walk, jump, run, or climb stairs. And perhaps most importantly of all, *the knee joint itself depends heavily on this muscle to stabilize it and support it as you're moving around all day long.*

Now at this point, some readers may be wondering, "What about the *other* knee muscles, aren't they important too?" Well, in this book we're going to primarily be concerned about strengthening just the quadriceps muscles–simply because it's the one that stands out among the others as being the main problem. For instance...

- 21 patients with symptomatic knee arthritis were compared to a control group of 21 people *without* knee pain (Hall 1993)

- all subjects had the strength of their quadriceps **and** hamstring muscles tested

- results showed that the arthritic knees had weaker quadriceps than the control group, *but not the hamstring muscles*

This is not an isolated finding either, as other studies have also found the quadriceps to be the "weakest link" of all the other knee muscles (Slemenda 1997).

Therefore, while it certainly wouldn't hurt anything to strengthen *every* single knee muscle, provided you have plenty of time and motivation, this book will just target the main problem muscle in knee arthritis, the quadriceps. After all, why use a bazooka when an arrow will do?

The *Correct* Way to Get Your Quadriceps Muscle in Shape

Okay, now that we know that most people with knee arthritis have weak quadriceps muscles, it's time to learn how to improve its function and make it *stronger*.

However before jumping right in and going over all the exercises you'll ever need to beef up your quadriceps, I think it's best to begin with a few strength training basics. Because I wrote this book with *everyone* in mind–from the athlete, to the retired person who just wants to be able to walk with their grandkids–it's only wise to make sure that we're all on the same page before going any further. Then, when we do get down to describing each of the strengthening exercises, *every* reader will know exactly what I mean when I say, "Do 1 set of 20 reps." So, using the handy question and answer format, let's start with the basics…

How do we make a muscle stronger?

Muscles get stronger only when we constantly challenge them to do more than they're used to doing. Do the same amount and type of activity over and over again, and your muscles will *never* increase in strength. For example, if Karen goes to the gym and lifts a ten-pound dumbbell up and down, ten times, workout after workout, week after week, her arms will *not* get any stronger by doing this exercise. Why? Because the human body is very efficient.

You see, right now, Karen's arm muscles can already do the job she is asking them to do (lift a ten-pound dumbbell ten times). Therefore, why should they bother growing any stronger? I mean after all, stronger, bigger muscles *do* require more calories, nutrition and maintenance from the body. And since they can *already* do everything they're asked to do, increasing in size and demanding more from the rest of the body would only be a waste of resources for no good reason.

It makes perfect sense if you stop and think about it, but we can also use this same line of thinking when it comes to making our muscles bigger and stronger– we simply *give* them a reason to get into better shape. And how do we do that? By simply asking them to do *more* than they're used to doing. Going back to the above example, if Karen wants make her arm muscles stronger, then she could maybe switch from a ten-pound dumbbell to a *twelve*-pound dumbbell the next time she goes to work out. Whoa! Her arm muscles won't be ready for that at all– they were always used to working with that ten-pound dumbbell. And so, they will have no choice but to get stronger now in order to meet the *new* demand Karen has placed on them.

For the more scientific-minded readers, the physiology textbooks call this *progressive resistance exercise.* You can use this very same strategy to get *any* muscle in your body stronger, and we're certainly going to be using it to get your quadriceps muscle as strong as we can.

What's the difference between a repetition and a set?

As we've said, we need to constantly challenge our muscles in order to force them to get stronger and one good way to do this is to lift a little heavier weight than we're used to using. Of course you won't always be able to lift a heavier and heavier weight *every* time you do an exercise, and so another option you have is to try to lift the same weight *more* times than you did before. As you can see, it's a good idea to keep track of things, just so you know for sure that you're actually making progress–which is where the terms "set" and "repetition" come into play.

If you take a weight and lift it up and down over your head once, you could say that you have just done one repetition or "rep" of that exercise. Likewise, if you take the same weight and lift it up and down a total of ten times over your head, then you could say that you did ten repetitions of that exercise.

A set, on the other hand, is simply a bunch of repetitions done one after the other. Using our above example once again, if you lifted a weight ten times over your head, and then rested, you would have just done one set of ten repetitions. Pretty straightforward isn't it?

Now the last thing you need to know about reps and sets is how we go about writing them down. The most common method used, is to first write the number of sets you did of an exercise, followed by an "x", and then the number of repetitions you did. For example, if you were able to lift a weight over your head ten times and then rested, you would write down 1x10. This means that you did 1 set of 10 repetitions of that particular exercise. Likewise, if the next workout you did 12 repetitions, you would write 1x12.

What's the best number of sets and repetitions to do
in order to make a muscle stronger?

There was a time when I asked myself that same question. So, in order to find out, I completely searched the published strength training literature starting from the year 1960. I then sorted out just the randomized controlled trials, since these provide the highest form of proof in medicine that something is really effective, and laid them all out on my kitchen table. While getting to that point took me literally months and months of daily reading and hunting down articles, it was really the only way I could come up with an accurate, evidence-based answer.

Now the first conclusion I came to was that it is quite possible for a person to get significantly stronger by doing any one of a *wide* variety of set and repetition combinations. For instance, one study might show that one set of eight to twelve repetitions could make a person stronger compared to a non-exercising control group–but then again so could four sets of thirteen to fifteen reps in another study.

Realizing this, I decided to change my strategy a bit and set my sights on finding the most *efficient* number of sets and repetitions. In other words, how many sets and repetitions could produce the best strength gains with the least amount of effort? And so, I had two issues to resolve. The first one was, "Are multiple sets of an exercise better than doing just one set?" and the second, "Exactly how many repetitions will produce the best strength gains?"

Anxious to get to the bottom of things, I returned once again to my pile of randomized controlled trials, this time searching for more specific answers. Here's what I found as far as sets are concerned:

- there are *many* randomized controlled trials showing that *one* set of an exercise is just as good as doing *three* sets of an exercise (Esquivel 2007, Starkey 1996, Reid 1987, Stowers 1983, Silvester 1982). This has been shown to be true in people who have just started weight training, as well in individuals that have been training for some time (Hass 2000).

Wow. With a lot of my patients either having limited time to exercise, or just plain hating it altogether, that was really good news. I could now tell them that based on strong evidence from many randomized controlled trials, all they needed to do was just *one set* of an exercise to get stronger–which would get them every bit as strong as doing three!

And the best number of repetitions to do? Well, that wasn't quite as cut and dried. The first thing I noted from the literature was that different numbers of repetitions have totally different training effects on the muscles. You see, it seems that the lower numbers of repetitions, say three or seven for example, train the muscles more for *strength*. On the other hand, the higher repetition numbers, such as twenty or twenty-five, tend to increase a muscle's *endurance* more than strength (endurance is where a muscle must repeatedly contract over and over for a long period of time such as when a person continuously moves their arms back and forth while vacuuming a rug for several minutes).

Another way to think about this is to simply imagine the repetition numbers sitting on a line. Repetitions that develop strength sit more toward the far left side of the line, and the number of repetitions that develop mainly endurance lie towards the right. Everything in the middle, therefore, would give you varying mixtures of both strength *and* endurance. The following is an example of this:

The Repetition Continuum

1 rep	10 reps	around 20 reps and higher

strength ———————————————————————— endurance ————————➔

Please note, however, that it's not like you won't gain *any* strength at all if you do an exercise for twenty repetitions or more. It's just that you'll gain mainly muscular endurance, and not near as much strength than if you would have done fewer repetitions (such as five or ten).

Okay, so now I knew there was a big difference between the lower repetitions and the higher repetitions. However one last question still stuck in my mind. Among the lower repetitions, are some better than others for gaining strength? For example, can I tell my patients that they will get stronger by doing a set of three or four repetitions as opposed to doing a set of nine or ten?

Well, it turns out that there really is no difference. For example, one randomized controlled trial had groups of exercisers do either three sets of 2-3 repetitions, three sets of 5-6 repetitions, or three sets of 9-10 repetitions (O'Shea 1966). After six weeks of training, everyone improved in strength, *with no significant differences among the three groups.*

And so, with this last piece of information, my lengthy (but profitable) investigation had finally come to an end. After scrutinizing some 45-plus years of strength training research, I could now make the following evidence-based conclusions:

- doing one set of an exercise is just as good as doing three sets of an exercise

- lower repetitions are best for building muscular strength, with no particular lower number being better than the others

- higher repetitions (around 20 or more) are best for building muscular *endurance*

In this book, we'll be taking full advantage of the above information by doing just one set of an exercise for ten to twenty repetitions. This means that you will use a weight that you can lift *at least* ten times in a row, and when you can lift it twenty times in good form, it's time to increase the weight a little to keep the progress going.

And why did I pick those numbers? Two reasons. The first has to do with the job of the quadriceps muscle. Since it plays a big role in stabilizing your knee, we want to boost its endurance and a long holding time the most. And this means we're going to lean a little more towards the *upper* repetitions in order to boost the endurance ability of the quadriceps, while still staying low enough to substantially increase its strength. Remember, from around the twenty repetitions mark and up, you're going to gain mostly muscular endurance and a lot less strength.

The second reason? Well, it's a matter of safety. Using higher repetitions enables us to not only gain plenty of strength, but also use much *lighter* weights than if we'd chosen to work with the lower repetitions. This is because it takes a much heavier weight to tire a muscle out in, say, five repetitions, than it does to tire a muscle out in fifteen. And since most people would agree that you have a better chance of injuring yourself with a heavier weight as opposed to a lighter one, I recommend leaning more towards the upper repetitions.

How many times a week do I have to do the exercises?

Doing the same strengthening exercise every day, or even five days a week will usually lead to overtraining–which means *no* strength gains. This is because the muscles need time to recover, which typically means at least a day or so in between exercise bouts to rest and rebuild before you stress 'em again. And so, the question then becomes, which is better, one, two or three times a week?

Well, believe it or not, when I went through the strength training literature in search of the optimal number of times a week to do a strengthening exercise, there were a few randomized controlled trials actually showing that doing a strengthening exercise *once* a week was just as good as doing it two or three times a week. However, these studies were done on *very* specific populations (such as the elderly) or *very* specific muscle groups that were worked in a special manner. Therefore, when you take this information, and couple it with the fact that there are a few randomized controlled trials showing that two and three times a week are far better than one time a week, there really isn't much support for the average person to do a strengthening exercise once a week to get stronger. And so, we're again left with another question of which is better, two versus three times a week–which is what much of the strength training research has investigated.

However it is at this point that the waters start to get a little muddy. If you take all the randomized controlled trials comparing two times a week to three times a week and lay them out on a table, you will get mixed results. In other words, there are some studies showing you that doing an exercise two times a week will get you the *same* results as three times a week, **but** there's also good research showing you that three times a week is *better* than two times a week. So what's one to do?

Well, in a case like this, the bottom line is that you can't really draw a firm conclusion one way or the other. So, you've got to work with what you've got. In this book, I'm going to recommend that you shoot for doing the strengthening exercises *three* times a week, because there is some good evidence that three times a week is better than two times a week (Braith 1989). However, I'm also going to add that if you have an unbelievably busy week, or just plain forget to do the exercises, I'll settle for two times a week because there is also substantial evidence that working out two times a week is just as good as working out three times a week (Carroll 1998, DeMichele 1997).

So there you have it. While it may have been a whole lot easier to just answer the question by saying "do the strengthening exercise two to three times a week," I think it's good for readers to know *exactly* why they're doing the things I'm suggesting *and* that there's a good, evidence-based reason behind it.

How hard should I push it when I do a set?

How hard you push yourself while doing an exercise, also known as *exercise intensity*, is another issue that certainly deserves mention and is a question I am frequently asked by patients. The answer lies in two pieces of information:

1. Doing an exercise until no further repetitions can be done in good form is called *momentary muscular failure*. Research shows us that getting to momentary muscular failure or close to it produces the best strength gains.

2. You should not be in pain while exercising.

Taking the above information into consideration, I feel that a person should keep doing an exercise as long as it isn't painful and until no further repetitions can be done in good form within the repetition scheme.

Does it make any difference how fast you do a repetition?

Many randomized controlled trials have shown that as far as gaining strength is concerned, it does *not* matter whether you do a repetition fast or slow (Berger 1966, Palmieri 1987, Young 1993). Here's a look at one of the studies:

- subjects were randomly divided into three groups (Berger 1966)

- each group did one set of the bench press exercise, which was performed in 25 seconds

- the first group did 4 repetitions in 25 seconds, the second group did 8-10 repetitions in 25 seconds, and the third did 18-20 repetitions in 25 seconds

- at the end of eight weeks, *there were no significant differences in the amount of strength gained between any of the groups*

So that's as far as strength is concerned. As far as safety, I recommend that you lift the weight up and down *smoothly* with each repetition, carefully avoiding any jerking motions.

What equipment will I need?

Since you'll be doing a strengthening exercise that involves lifting weights, it's a no brainer you're going to need something to lift. Remember from our discussion on pages 32 and 33 that muscles get stronger only when we constantly challenge them to do more than they're used to doing. So, this means that taking the same weight, and lifting it over and over again, week after week, simply won't get the job done. Therefore, you'll need to have *several* weights of varying pounds available to use.

Now if you think this will involve a lot of money, it doesn't have to. By far, the easiest and cheapest way to go is to buy a set of *adjustable* ankle weights. You can get them at most sporting good stores and they typically look something like this:

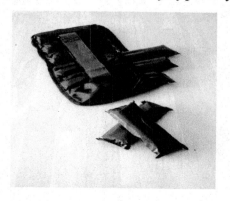

As you can see from the picture, the cuff can attach quite easily to your ankle by means of a velcro strap. Also note that the cuff is made up of six mini weight packs that you can take in and out of their little pockets, depending on how many pounds you want to use. Since the cuff in the picture weighs a total of 10 pounds, and has six little packs, this means that each one weighs a little over a pound and a half. This allows you to increase the weight *gradually* on any given exercise–which is one of the biggest advantages of using *adjustable* cuff weights.

Some tips on buying them. First, be aware that there are *wrist* cuffs and there are *ankle* cuffs (the above picture shows an ankle cuff). Wrist cuffs are smaller, but I recommend getting the ankle cuffs, mainly because they are heavier which allows you to go up higher in weight over time than the wrist cuffs. Second, pay particular attention to how many total pounds *each cuff* weighs. How much weight should you look for? Probably two 10-pound cuffs will give you a good workout for awhile. If the need arises, they do make two 20-pound cuffs which are also widely available.

As far as cost, I have priced these cuffs at a lot of places and the average cost is around twenty dollars for a pair–not a bad investment considering one pair should last for years with normal use.

The only other equipment you *might* need are some dumbbells. One of the exercises involves holding a weight in each hand, and if you're not able to grasp the cuff weights or attach them to your wrists, then a pair of dumbbells will work. Once again, the easiest thing to do is to just go to a sporting goods store (or large retail store), and purchase several light dumbbells. Most look something like this:

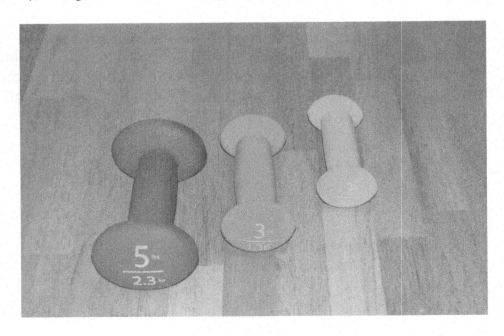

Light dumbbells such as these are inexpensive, which is a good thing, because you're going to need to get several different sizes as you progress with the exercise program. Of course you technically can use any kind of weight that's comfortable to grip and allows you to progress to a heavier weight in small increments.

How much weight should I start off with?

For reasons we've discussed earlier in this chapter, I recommend you shoot for doing one set of an exercise for ten to twenty repetitions. Therefore, you should start out with a weight that allows you to do a minimum of ten repetitions, but no more than twenty. But how do you figure that out?

Well, by a little trial and error. The first time you do a particular exercise, you're just going to have to take your best guess at how much weight will allow you to do between 10 and 20 repetitions, try the exercise, and then see how it goes. As an example, say you're going to try a quadriceps exercise and you decide to fill the cuff weight up with five pounds, begin lifting it, and find you can do 15 repetitions in good form. That's great–you've hit our target range of 10 to 20 reps! Next time, you'll use five pounds again, and try and do a few more reps, eventually working up to 20 reps before adding more weight.

The other thing that commonly happens when you're doing an exercise for the first time, is that you might find it's either too heavy (maybe you could lift it only once or twice) *or* it's way too light (maybe you could lift it twenty-five times or more). Here again, that's not a big problem. When trying the exercise the next time, simply take another good guess and adjust the weight up or down a little as needed. Do keep in mind that when *anyone* starts a weight training program, or tries a new exercise for the first time, it's perfectly normal for it to take one or two exercise sessions to find the appropriate weight.

Like I said, it'll be a matter of a little trial and error at first, but do keep in mind that when it comes to strengthening your quads, the main idea is not to see how much weight you can lift, but rather to find a safe starting weight, and then *gradually progress* over time.

A Quick Note on *Isometric* Exercise

The guidelines you've just read about apply to those type of strengthening exercises where your muscles contract while you're lifting a weight up and down. In exercise science, this type of exercise is known as *isotonic* exercise.

However what does one do if they need to strengthen their quadriceps, *but they can barely move their knee at all?* Well if this is you, then rest easy. There is yet another proven way to strengthen the quadriceps that involves very little knee motion. Impossible you say? Not really. It's called *isometric* exercise.

The word *isometric* comes from the two Greek words *isos*, meaning "equal" or "like," and *metron*, meaning measure. An isometric exercise, then, is one in which the length of the muscle stays the same as it is contracting. A good example of this is when you use your hand and arm to push hard against a brick wall. Your arm is still and unable to move because you can't push the wall over, yet, there is a definite building up of tension in your muscles that can be used as a type of resistance exercise.

But can something so simple as pushing on an immovable object *really* make one stronger? You bet it can or it wouldn't be in this book. Here are a couple of studies that may surprise a few readers...

- 20 subjects were randomly assigned to either an exercise group or a control group (Carolan 1992)

- those in the exercise group did 30 isometric contractions of their quadriceps muscles per a day, three days a week, for 8 weeks

- the control group did not exercise

- results showed that only those subjects that did the isometric exercise increased the strength of their quadriceps muscle by a whopping 33%

and…

- 15 subjects were randomly assigned to either an exercise group or a control group (Garfinkel 1992)

- those in the exercise group did 30 isometric contractions of their quadriceps muscles per a day, three days a week, for 8-weeks

- the control group did not exercise

- all subjects had CT scans taken of their mid-thigh to see if their muscles had gotten any bigger

- researchers found that after 8-weeks, those subjects who did the isometric exercise had quadriceps muscles that were 15% *bigger* and 28% *stronger*!

With proof that isometrics can *truly* make a person's quadriceps bigger and stronger, it's just the perfect type of strengthening exercise for those readers who have such a painful knee that they can hardly bend or move it around at all.

So what exactly does isometric exercise involve anyway? Well, not much. The exercise in this book merely requires a person to put their knee in a specific position, and then push down against a rolled-up pillow. Pretty easy, huh?

Now as far as how long and how many times you push, as well as how often, we'll once again be using evidence-based guidelines taken straight from multiple randomized controlled trials which have proven that isometrics can truly increase muscle size and strength. They are:

- push as hard as you comfortably can for 3-5 seconds
- repeat for a total of 30 times, once a day
- do this three times a week

And with this last bit of strength-training information, we're finished discussing the basics. So, now that we're all on the same page, let's move on to some of the best quadriceps strengthening exercises medical research has to offer…

Isometric Quadriceps Exercise

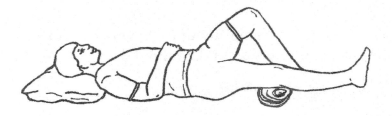

- get into the position as the above picture. You can either recline on your elbows or lie flat on your back.

- fold a pillow in half, and place it under the knee of the leg that is straight, as shown. If this doesn't feel right, you can do the exercise without the pillow, with your knee straight.

- press down as hard as you comfortably can into the pillow with the knee that is straight, and hold for 3-5 seconds. The muscle on the top of your leg, above the kneecap (the quadriceps), should tighten up.

- do this 30 times in a row, once a day

- repeat the exercise three times a week, separated by a day of rest in between sessions (either Monday-Wednesday-Friday or Tuesday-Thursday-Saturday)

- if necessary, work up to the 30 repetitions by adding a few more reps each session until your reach 30

Chair Leg Extension Exercise

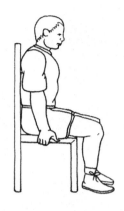 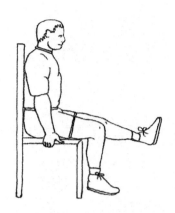 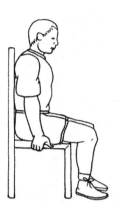

Starting Position   **Midpoint**   **Finish Position**

- sit in a stationary chair with your back supported as in the starting position

- holding on to the chair as needed, kick your leg out as straight as is comfortably possible like the middle picture–*but do not lock it out completely* . If you can only kick your leg out just a little, that's okay. In time, as you have less pain and become stronger and more flexible, you will be able to kick it out farther.

- hold for 1-2 seconds (as in middle picture), and then slowly lower your leg to the floor

- do this 20 times in a row, once a day

- repeat the exercise three times a week, separated by a day of rest in between sessions (either Monday-Wednesday-Friday or Tuesday-Thursday-Saturday)

- if necessary, work up to the 20 repetitions by adding a few more reps each session until you reach 20 in a row

- start out with no weight, and when you can do 20 reps in good form, add a pound or two with your ankle weights

Leg Extension Machine

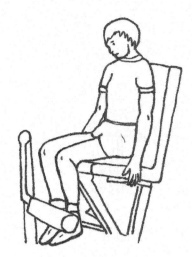

Readers who have access to a gym that has weight machines can substitute the chair leg extension exercise on the last page for the *leg extension machine*. This is because the knee motion is the same, and so it still works the quadriceps muscle. While leg extension machines can vary a bit from place to place, they all look similar to the one in the above picture.

Since it is important that the leg extension machine's seat be adjusted appropriately to each individual, it is suggested that the reader consult with knowledgeable staff at their gym facility to help them set the seat and learn how to use the machine correctly. Know that if you do choose to use the leg extension machine instead of the chair leg extension exercise, the same exercise guidelines still apply…

- start off with a weight that allows you to do at least 10 repetitions, but no more than 20

- work up to 20 repetitions. When you can do 20 reps in good form, add some weight.

- do only one set per session

- repeat the exercise three times a week, separated by a day of rest in between sessions (either Monday-Wednesday-Friday or Tuesday-Thursday-Saturday)

Chair Squat Exercise

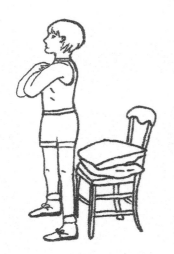 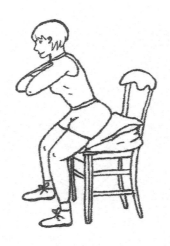 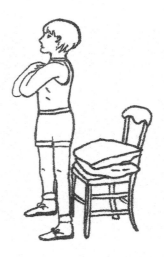

Starting Position **Midpoint** **Finish Position**

- find a sturdy chair, put a pillow or two in it, and stand in front of it like you're going to sit down. You should be in the starting position.

- keeping your back straight and bending at the hips, slowly sit down in the chair as in the middle picture. As soon as your buttocks touch the pillow, immediately start coming back up to the standing position. If you have poor balance, make sure that you have someone next to you for safety.

- do this 20 times in a row, once a day

- repeat the exercise three times a week, separated by a day of rest in between sessions (either Monday-Wednesday-Friday or Tuesday-Thursday-Saturday)

- if necessary, work up to the 20 repetitions by adding a few more reps each session until your reach 20 in a row

- The progression goes like this. When you can do 20 reps in good form with 2 pillows, use 1. When you can do 20 reps in good form with 1 pillow, use no pillow. If you can do 20 reps in good form with no pillow, try doing it with a light dumbbell in each hand, say 5 pounds, and increase the weight as needed.

Leg Press Machine

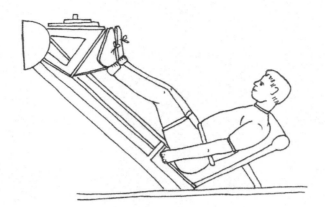

Readers who have access to a gym that has weight machines can substitute the chair squat exercise on the last page for the *leg press machine*. This is because the knee motion is the same, and so it still works the quadriceps muscle. While leg press machines can vary a bit from place to place, for instance some may sit more horizontally on the floor, they all look similar to the one above in that you are sitting down and pushing out with both your legs.

Since it is important that the leg press machine be adjusted appropriately to each individual, it is suggested that the reader consult with knowledgeable staff at their gym facility to help them set the seat and learn how to use the machine correctly. Know that if you do choose to use the leg press machine instead of the chair squat exercise, the same exercise guidelines still apply…

- start off with a weight that allows you to do at least 10 repetitions, but no more than 20
- work up to 20 repetitions. When you can do 20 reps in good form, add some weight.
- do only one set per session
- repeat the exercise three times a week, separated by a day of rest in between sessions (either Monday-Wednesday-Friday or Tuesday-Thursday-Saturday)

Alright. I've just shown you *five* exercise that will without a doubt strengthen your quadriceps muscle. So which ones do you have to do? Well, be rest assured you don't have to do *all* of them.

If you have a lot of pain and can hardly move your knee much, start out with the *isometric quadriceps exercise...*

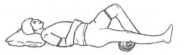

If you can tolerate kicking your leg out, just do the *chair leg extension exercise* and the *chair squat exercise...*

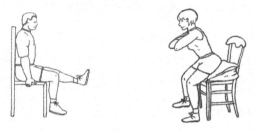

If you have access to a gym, just do the *leg extension machine* and the *leg press machine...*

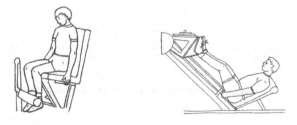

Towards the end of the book (Chapter 7), we'll put the quadriceps exercises together with all the other exercises in the book for one simple weekly routine. For now, just get familiar with the exercises. Let's move on now to Tune-Up #2...

Quick Review

✓ many studies point out that people with knee arthritis have weak quadriceps muscles, a key stabilizer of the knee joint

✓ in order for muscles to get stronger, they must be progressively challenged with more weight

✓ multiple randomized controlled trials point out that muscles can be adequately strengthened by doing just one set of an exercise to momentary muscular failure

✓ lower repetitions have a tendency to increase a muscle's *strength,* while higher repetitions (around 20 or more) have more of a tendency to increase a muscle's *endurance*

✓ randomized controlled trials show that strengthening exercises should be done two to three times a week in order to make a muscle stronger

✓ randomized controlled trials also reveal that isometric exercise is capable of significantly increasing a muscle's size and strength by contracting the muscle as hard as is comfortably possible for 3-5 seconds, thirty times a day, three days a week.

Tune-Up #2:
How to Make Your Knee *More* Flexible

So far we've talked about restoring your knees muscular *strength*. While critically important, it's still only one piece of the puzzle when it comes to treating your arthritis by improving the function of your knee. Why? Because the strongest muscles in the world will do you little good if all you can do is move your knee back and forth a few degrees!

And this brings us to the issue of *flexibility*, or what physical therapists call *range on motion*. While it makes sense that a well-functioning knee should have good range of motion, I never add another exercise to a patient's already busy day unless I've got a good evidence-based reason to do so. Having said that, let's see what the research has to say about the flexibility of people with knee arthritis…

- 54 people with knee arthritis were compared to 53 age and sex matched control subjects *without* knee arthritis (Liikavainio 2008)

- researchers measured how much subjects could bend their knees

- it was found that on average, those with knee arthritis could bend their knees 14 degrees *less* than those with no knee arthritis

---

and

- 15 people with painful knee arthritis were compared to 15 control subjects (matched by age, mass, and gender) with *no* knee pain (Messier 1992)

- researchers measured how much subjects could bend and straighten their knees

- results showed that those with knee arthritis could bend and straighten their knees *significantly less* than the control subjects with no pain

---

As the studies reveal, people with knee arthritis tend to have *really* poor knee flexibility. No need to worry though, that's a problem we intend to tackle right now…

Stretching Secrets That Work

While there are many different techniques to choose from when it comes to stretching out a tight muscle, by far the easiest and least complicated way is known as *the static stretch*. A static (or stationary) stretch takes a tight muscle, puts it in a lengthened position, and keeps it there for a certain period of time. For instance, if you wanted to use the static stretch technique to make your back muscles more flexible, you could simply lie on your back and pull your knees to your chest. Thus, as you are holding this position, the back muscles are being *statically stretched*. There's no bouncing, just a gentle, sustained stretch.

It sounds easy, perhaps a bit *too* easy, so you may be wondering at this point just how effective static stretching really is when it comes to making one more flexible. Well, a quick review of the stretching research pretty much lays it out straight as there are *multiple* randomized controlled trials clearly in agreement that this is a winning method. Here are the highlights…

- a study published in the journal *Physical Therapy* took 57 subjects and randomly divided them up into four groups (Bandy 1994)

- the first group held their static stretch for a length of 15 seconds, the second group for 30 seconds, and the third for 60. The fourth group (the control group) did not stretch at all.

- all three groups performed *one* stretch a day, five days a week, for six weeks

- results showed that holding a stretch for a period of 30 seconds was just as effective at increasing flexibility as holding one for 60 seconds. Also, holding a stretch for a period of 30 seconds was much more effective than holding one for 15 seconds or (of course) not stretching at all.

Hmm. Looks like if you hold a stretch for 15 seconds, it doesn't do much to make you more flexible. On the other hand, holding a stretch for 30 full seconds *does* work–and just as well as 60 seconds!

Wow. So now that we know 30 seconds seems to be the magic number, makes you wonder if doing *a bunch* of 30-second stretches would be *even better* than doing it one time a day like they did in the study…

- another randomized controlled trial done several years later (Bandy 1997) set out to research not only the optimal length of time to hold a static stretch, *but also the optimal number of times to do it*

- 93 subjects were recruited and randomly placed into one of five groups: 1) perform three 1-minute stretches; 2) perform three 30-second stretches; 3) perform a 1-minute stretch; 4) perform a 30-second stretch; or 5) do no stretching at all (the control group)

- the results? Not so surprising was the fact that all groups that stretched became more flexible than the control group that didn't stretch.

- however what *was* surprising was the finding that among the groups that did stretch, no one group became more flexible than the other!

- in other words, the researchers found that as far as trying to become more flexible, it made no difference whether the stretching time was increased from 30 to 60 seconds, OR when the frequency was changed from doing one stretch a day to doing three stretches a day

So here we have yet *another* randomized controlled trial (the kind of study that provides the highest form of proof in medicine) which is showing us once again that holding a stretch for 30 seconds is *just as effective* as holding it for 60 seconds. And to top it all off, doing the 30-second stretch *once* a day is just as good as if you did it three times!

Interestingly, other randomized controlled trials have also supported the effectiveness of the 30-second stretch done one time a day, five days a week, to make one more flexible (Bandy 1998). Fantastic!

So as the randomized controlled trials *clearly* point out, it really doesn't take a lot of time to stretch out tight muscles *if* you know how. Based on the current published stretching research, this book recommends the following guidelines for the average person needing to stretch out a tight muscle with the static stretch technique:

- get into the starting position
- next, begin moving into the stretch position until a *gentle* stretch is felt
- once this position is achieved, hold for a full 30 seconds
- when the 30 seconds is up, *slowly* release the stretch
- do this one time a day, five days a week

One last note. While it is acceptable to feel a little discomfort while doing a stretch, it is *not* okay to be in pain. Do not force yourself to get into any stretching position, and by all means, skip the stretch entirely if it makes your pain worse.

The Three Motions of Your Knee

Okay. Now that you know how to make your knee more flexible, we need to talk about which knee motions need to be improved the most. So how many different ways does your knee move anyway?

Well, while most people think of your knee as only being able to swing back and forth like a door hinge, the truth is that your knee actually *rotates* as well. Although this may seem a bit unbelievable, the truth is that with each step you take, your lower leg bone (the tibia) actually rotates *outward*. On the next page is a neat little test you can do that demonstrates this little-known knee motion...

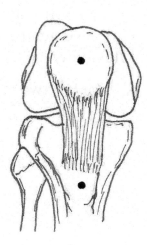

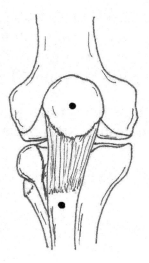

Figure 20. What the right knee looks like from the front when your knee is *bent*. Note that the dots are in line with each other.

Figure 21. What the right knee looks like from the front when your knee is *straight*. Note that the lower dot has moved to the side.

- to try the above test, sit down *with your knee bent at a right angle*. Then, take a pen and put a dot in the middle of your kneecap (top dot).

- next, put another mark on the bony bump that sticks out on the lower leg just below your kneecap (lower dot)

- make sure the dots are in line with each other as in Figure 20

- now, while still sitting, kick your leg out

- your knee should now be straight and the dots should look like Figure 21

- note that the dots are no longer in a straight line. This is because your lower leg bone has rotated *outward* as you straightened your leg. This same motion also occurs as you are walking.

Pretty nifty test, huh? I discovered that one years ago in an old book I came across while I was digging around in the medical library. Now if you did discover that your knee was too tight to do the test, don't worry, the stretching exercises in this chapter can most certainly help you regain normal flexibility.

Okay, so that's *one* of the three major knee motions. The last two are *extension*, which is the motion of straightening your knee…

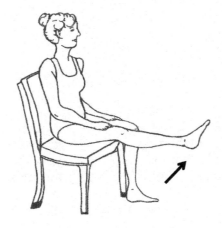

Figure 22. A person with her right knee in extension. The motion of extension is when one is *straightening* their knee.

and *flexion*, which is when you're bending your knee…

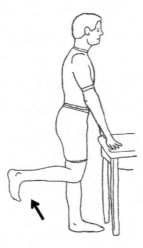

Figure 23. A person with his right knee in flexion. The motion of flexion is when one is *bending* their knee.

The Two Stretches That Will Get the Job Done

Okay, time for the meat and potatoes of the chapter–the stretches! To date, the knee motions that have been found to be restricted the most in people with arthritis are knee *flexion* and *extension*. Therefore, this means that there are two main muscle groups that we need to be concerned about the most when it comes to restoring knee motion. They are:

- *the quadriceps muscles*. Put your hand on the front of your thigh and you'll be right on them. If they're tight, they can keep you from being able to bend your leg back to your buttocks. Therefore, stretching them will improve your knee *flexion*.

- *the hamstrings muscles*. If you put your hand on the back of your thigh, you're right on these muscles. If they're tight, they can keep your leg from straightening your leg out all the way. Therefore, stretching them out will improve your knee *extension*.

Since no one stretch will work for every single reader, I will be showing you two stretches for the hamstrings and two for the quadriceps–so just pick the one from each muscle group that is the easiest for you to do.

In case you're wondering, they're all equally effective, provided you use the evidence-based stretching guidelines we covered earlier in the chapter. On the next few pages are the stretches…

Quadriceps Stretch #1

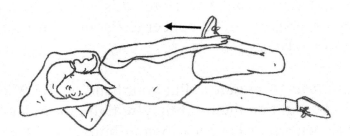

1. Get into the same position as the above picture. It's okay to be on a bed or on the floor.

2. Grab your ankle and pull your foot backward toward your buttocks until you feel a gentle stretch in the *front* of your thigh.

3. You can bring your knee backward for an even stronger stretch.

4. Hold for 30 full seconds.

5. Do this once a day, five days a week. It's okay to work up to the 30 seconds if you have to.

Quadriceps Stretch #2

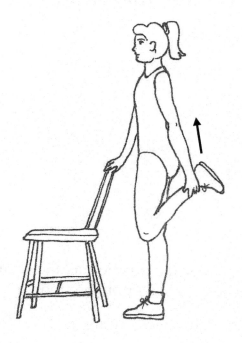

1. Get into the same position as the above picture. Use a sturdy chair or perhaps a countertop.

2. Grab your ankle and pull your foot backward toward your buttocks until you feel a gentle stretch in the *front* of your thigh.

3. You can bring your knee backward for an even stronger stretch.

4. Hold for 30 full seconds.

5. Do this once a day, five days a week. It's okay to work up to the 30 seconds if you have to.

Hamstring Stretch #1

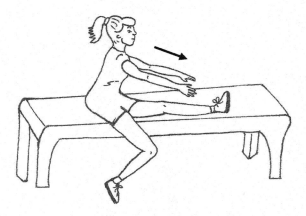

1. Get into the same position as the above picture. It's okay to be on a bed or on the floor.

2. Keeping your back straight, lean forward toward your foot until you feel a gentle stretch on the *back* of your thigh. Try to bend forward from the hips as much as possible, rather than bending from your low back.

3. Try to keep your knee straight.

4. Hold for 30 full seconds.

5. Do this once a day, five days a week. It's okay to work up to the 30 seconds if you have to.

Hamstring Stretch #2

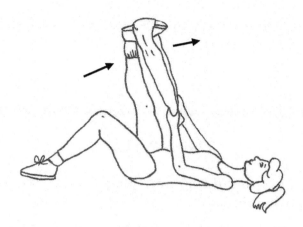

1. Using a towel, get into the above position. It's okay to be on a bed or on the floor.

2. Pull your foot toward you until you feel a gentle stretch in the *back* of your thigh.

3. Try to keep your knee straight.

4. Hold for 30 full seconds.

5. Do this once a day, five days a week. It's okay to work up to the 30 seconds if you have to.

Pretty simple stretches, huh? By applying the evidence-based guidelines to the stretches, you will be sending a clear signal to your muscles that they need to elongate and stretch out. Then, over a period of weeks, the tissues will begin to gradually lengthen bit by bit–which means *more* flexibility for your knee. And improved function equals less pain…

Quick Review

✓ many studies have found that patients with knee arthritis have decreased knee flexibility

✓ one of the easiest and most effective ways of becoming more flexible is to use the *static stretching* technique

✓ according to randomized controlled trials, holding a static stretch for 15 seconds does little to increase one's flexibility. On the other hand, holding a static stretch for 30 seconds is just as effective as holding one for 60 seconds.

✓ randomized controlled trials also point out that doing one 30-second static stretch is just as effective as doing *three* 30-second static stretches

✓ additionally, randomized controlled trials have shown that doing your static stretching exercises five times a week is quite sufficient to make your muscles longer

---

Tune-Up #3:
How to Improve Your
Proprioception

Pronounced pro-pree-o-ception, all this fourteen-letter word means is the ability you have at any given moment to sense the position and movements of your body. For example, if you close your eyes, you could probably tell me without much difficulty if your elbows are bent or straight, or if your head is turned to the left or right–all without even looking.

To give you more of an idea of just how critical proprioception is, here are a few everyday activities whose success or failure depends on the proper functioning of your sense of *proprioception…*

- getting something out of your pocket
- pushing down on the gas or brake pedal in your car
- walking in the dark
- scratching that hard-to-reach spot on your back

As you can see, all of these activities involve doing something without the help of your vision. By giving your brain constant updates as to the position of your body parts, your proprioception helps you out a lot when you are unable to see exactly what you are doing.

Over the years, researchers have tested the proprioception of people with knee arthritis–and guess what they're finding…

- 77 people with painful knee arthritis were compared to 63 people with no knee pain (Hassan 2001)

- proprioception was tested by moving the leg to a certain angle, holding it there for 5 seconds, returning it to the original position, and then asking subjects to reproduce the test angle. This was done with the subject's eyes closed.

- testing showed that those with painful knee arthritis had significantly reduced proprioception compared to those with no knee pain and…

- 117 patients with advanced knee arthritis that were scheduled for knee replacement surgery were compared to 40 subjects with no pain or knee arthritis (Koralewicz 2000)

- the researchers tested everybody's proprioception

- interestingly, those scheduled for knee replacements had significantly reduced proprioception compared to those with no arthritis or pain

---

These studies clearly show us that *many* people with painful knee arthritis have much difficulty sensing the positions and movements of their knees correctly. So the next question is, can this delicate sense be restored? Let's take a look…

- researchers studied a group of patients with knee arthritis that were 50 to 70 years old (Tsauo 2008)

- patients were randomized into two groups. One group, a training group, did specific proprioception exercises, while a control group did not.

- all subjects had the proprioception sense in their knees tested before and after the study

- after 8-weeks, those that did the proprioception exercises had significantly increased their knee proprioception compared to the control group

---

Studies conducted like the one above bring us good news–proprioception sense *can* be improved in the knees of people with arthritis, in a matter of *weeks* no less, a finding that has been duplicated over and over (Jan 2009 and Hurley 1998).

Once again, we sit here having identified yet *another* functional loss in arthritic knees–decreased proprioception–and have a good tool to restore it. Having said that, this next exercise is designed to specifically do just that…

Knee Proprioception Exercise

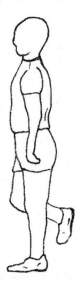

1. Stand on one leg in the same position as the above picture. Your knee can be straight or slightly bent, whichever is more comfortable.

2. If you can't balance well on one leg at all, or if you feel like you might fall, stand next to a table, chair, or doorway–something you can lightly hold on to.

3. Try to stay standing on one leg for 30 full seconds.

4. When you can stand on one leg, well-balanced, for 30 full seconds *without holding on to anything,* it's time to make it more challenging by closing your eyes.

5. When you can stand on one leg, well balanced, for 30 full seconds, without holding on to anything *and your eyes closed,* you can try for 60 seconds for an advanced challenge.

6. If you find you simply cannot stand on one leg without holding on to something, that's okay, just follow the same progression above, except hold on as lightly as you safely can.

A few comments about this exercise. Number one, it's much harder than it looks. If at first glance you're thinking, "That looks too easy" –give it a try. If you can stand on one leg, well balanced, for 60 full seconds with your eyes closed, you can skip it as far as I'm concerned.

And how often do you need to do it? Well, since there's little research telling us how often a person needs to do this exercise to get *the best* results, I recommend doing it three times a week with a day of rest in between, just as with the quadriceps strengthening exercises. Week-by-week, the exercise will begin to get easier and easier, indicating that you're well on your way to improving your proprioception.

Quick Review

✓ **proprioception is your ability to sense the position and movements of your body**

✓ **studies show that many people with knee arthritis have abnormal proprioception in their knee joints**

✓ **studies have also proven that this lost proprioception can be improved in a matter of weeks**

Tune-Up #4:
How to Improve Knee
Endurance

If I ended the book right now, you'd have exercises that would make your knee stronger, more flexible, and more responsive. While this may sound good enough, it still leaves out one last function a knee absolutely has to have–*endurance*. For without endurance, your knee wouldn't let you do simple things like walk for very long at all.

So what exactly is endurance? Well, in simple terms, it's your ability to do something over and over again, repeatedly, for a long period of time. Crack open a physiology book, however, and you'll get a little different story. Basically there are two types of endurance, and they're both important to know about when it comes to your knee arthritis.

The first is called *cardiovascular endurance*, or as I like to call it "whole body" endurance. This is the ability your body has to do something over and over again, and usually involves several large muscle groups. Going out walking or riding a bike for an hour or so are a few examples–these activities involve repeated contractions of *many* muscles, and work your heart as well. Here's what researchers have found when they've checked out the cardiovascular endurance of people with knee arthritis…

> • one study looked at 18 patients with knee arthritis that were waiting to have knee replacements. They were compared to 18 age and sex-matched controls with no knee pain (Philbin 1995).
>
> • all subjects took a cardiovascular endurance test which involved measuring how much oxygen they used as they exercised
>
> • the knee arthritis patients were found to be *significantly* deconditioned compared to the control group with no knee pain

As this study shows us, if you have knee arthritis and find that you lack "stamina" when you get out and do things, well, you're clearly not alone.

So that's *cardiovascular* endurance. The second type of endurance is known as *muscular* endurance. This is the ability of a single muscle (or muscle group) to contract over and over. A good example of this is sitting in a chair and kicking your leg out for ten minutes. Unlike walking or running, which involves a bunch of muscles, kicking your leg out would mainly be an endurance activity for just your quadriceps muscle. Here again, the research has pinpointed more problems…

- 45 men and 45 women with knee arthritis were compared to 41 males and 63 females with no knee pain (Fisher 1997)

- in this study, researchers specifically tested the endurance of the quadriceps and hamstring muscles individuallly

- it was found that those subjects with knee arthritis had significantly lower endurance of both their quadriceps and hamstring muscles compared to those with no knee pain

---

Apparently people with knee arthritis have *a lot* of problems with endurance. But, that's okay, because decreased endurance is yet another missing knee function that we can most certainly get back over a period of *weeks* (Kovar 1992, Talbot 2003). And now I'm going to show you how.

On the following pages are *five* of the best and easiest ways for you to increase the endurance of your knee muscles. Also know that since these activities involve the contraction of many large muscles (like your quadriceps) your heart and cardiovascular system will get a workout as well–which addresses the problem of decreased cardiovascular endurance so commonly found in people with knee arthritis.

Keep in mind that you only need to do *one* endurance exercise to increase your cardiovascular and muscular endurance, so just pick the one you like the best. Remember too that you can always alternate them, or switch them from time-to-time to keep from becoming bored.

Endurance Exercise #1

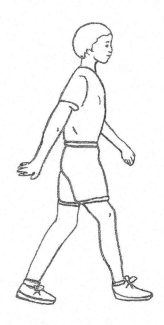

Simple enough, the first endurance exercise is *walking*. Since it involves contracting the quadriceps and hamstring muscles over and over, it will most certainly increase both your muscular, as well as your cardiovascular endurance. And perhaps best of all, it requires no special equipment because all you need is, well, some space! To get the endurance benefits of walking, follow these simple guidelines…

- Walk at a comfortable pace. To build endurance, the key isn't so much how fast your legs are moving, but that you *keep* them moving.

- Go for time, not distance. Your goal should be to work up to 20 to 30 minutes of continuous walking, 2-3 times a week. It really doesn't matter if you can only make it 1 minute or 10 minutes the first time you go walking–the next time shoot for walking a minute or two *more* if possible. By adding time bit-by-bit, you'll soon be up to our target of walking for a full 20 to 30 minutes.

Endurance Exercise #2

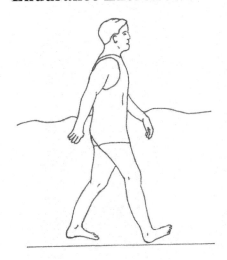

Pool walking is the next endurance exercise. It offers the same benefits as walking on land, except it has one big advantage–the water supports your body, which allows you to exercise with *less* weight on your knees. In fact, I've actually had patients who couldn't walk on land, but could in the water! To get the endurance benefits of walking in pool, follow these guidelines…

- Walk at a comfortable pace. To build endurance, the key isn't so much how fast your legs are moving, but that you *keep* them moving.

- Go for time, not distance. Your goal should be to work up to 20 to 30 minutes of continuous walking, 2-3 times a week. It really doesn't matter if you can only make it 1 minute or 10 minutes the first time you go walking–the next time shoot for walking a minute or two *more* if possible. By adding time bit-by-bit, you'll soon be up to our target of walking for a full 20 to 30 minutes.

- Know too that the higher the water is, the less weight and stress there will be on your knees. For example, when the water is up to your waist, you're at approximately 50% of your true body weight, and when the water is up to your chest, you're at approximately 25% of your true body weight. Pretty neat!

Endurance Exercise #3

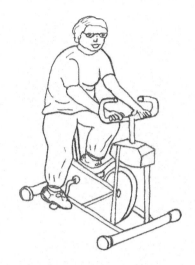

The *exercise bike* offers us yet another way to increase the endurance of our knee muscles. Like walking in a pool, the exercise bike has the advantage of working your knee with less body weight on it. To get the endurance benefits of the exercise bike, follow these guidelines...

- Make sure the seat height is adjusted correctly! A seat that is too low will cause your knee to bend too much and create problems. On the other hand, a seat that is too high can be uncomfortable because it leaves you "reaching" for the pedal. Therefore, set the seat height so that your knee is comfortable as your foot goes *all* the way around the pedal cycle.

- Once you've set the seat height correctly, make sure the bike is set on the *least* amount of resistance.

- Now you're set–start pedaling and go for time. Your goal should be to work up to 20 to 30 minutes of continuous pedaling, 2-3 times a week. It really doesn't matter if you can only make it 1 minute or 10 minutes the first time you try–the next time shoot for pedaling a minute or two *more* if possible. By adding time bit-by-bit, you'll soon be up to our target of pedaling for a full 20 to 30 minutes. After you can do 20 to 30 minutes on the least amount of resistance, you can bump the resistance up a notch and build back up to 20 to 30 minutes again for an added challenge.

Endurance Exercise #4

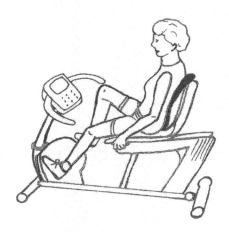

Endurance Exercise #4 is the *recumbent bike*. It offers the same benefits as the exercise bike on the last page, except it has one big advantage–the seat has a back that supports your spine–a big plus for those with back pain. Being that it's still an exercise bike, the same guidelines still apply…

- Make sure the seat is adjusted correctly! The seats on these recumbent bikes *slide* back and forth, unlike the previous exercise bike where the seats adjust up and down. If you have the seat too far forward, it will cause your knees to bend too much and create problems. On the other hand, a seat that is too far back can be uncomfortable because it leaves you "reaching" for the pedal. Therefore, set the seat so that your knee is comfortable as your foot goes *all* the way around the pedal cycle.

- Once you've set the seat correctly, make sure the bike is set on the *least* amount of resistance.

- Now you're set–start pedaling and go for time. Your goal should be to work up to 20 to 30 minutes of continuous pedaling, 2-3 times a week. It really doesn't matter if you can only make it 1 minute or 10 minutes the first time you try–the next time shoot for pedaling a minute or two *more* if possible. By adding time bit-by-bit, you'll soon be up to our target of pedaling for a full 20 to 30 minutes. After you can do 20 to 30 minutes on the least amount of resistance, you can bump the resistance up a notch and build back up to 20 to 30 minutes again for an added challenge.

Endurance Exercise #5

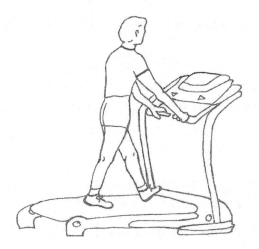

The last endurance exercise is the *treadmill*. Of course it's really walking, except there are a few advantages. First, you can use a treadmill even when the weather is bad outside–a definite advantage over walking outdoors. Second, treadmills force you to keep walking at a fixed pace, since the belt under your feet keeps moving which makes you go as fast as the treadmill does. To get the endurance benefits of the treadmill, follow these guidelines…

- Start out with the treadmill *flat*. Whether you choose to hold on to the handles or swing your arms freely depends on how good your balance is.

- Set the treadmill to a comfortable speed. Remember, to build endurance, the key isn't how fast your legs are moving, but that you *keep* them moving.

- Once again, go for time. Your goal should be to work up to 20 to 30 minutes of continuous walking, 2-3 times a week. It really doesn't matter if you can only make it 1 minute or 10 minutes the first time you go walking–the next time shoot for walking a minute or two *more* if possible. By adding time bit-by-bit, you'll soon be up to our target of walking for a full 20 to 30 minutes. After you can do 20 to 30 minutes at a comfortable speed, you can increase the speed a bit and build back up to 20 to 30 minutes again for an added challenge.

> ## *Quick Review*
>
> ✓ *cardiovascular endurance* is the ability your body has to do something over and over again, and usually involves several large muscle groups
>
> ✓ *muscular endurance* is the ability of a single muscle (or muscle group) to contract repeatedly
>
> ✓ studies show that many people with knee arthritis have decreased cardiovascular *and* muscular endurance
>
> ✓ studies have also demonstrated that these decreases in endurance can be improved in a matter of weeks

Putting It All Together:
The Six-Week Program

The first exercise program I ever wrote for publication consisted of three exercises, and I asked the reader to choose *only one.* The exercises were shown to be effective in randomized controlled trials, and if the diligent reader truly followed my specific, evidence-based guidelines, I could all but guarantee that their pain would improve, if not go away altogether.

Eventually the book was translated into other languages, and as its popularity grew, I started getting some interesting feedback from worldwide readers. Two points consistently came up regarding this exercise routine:

- there weren't enough exercises in the book

- the exercises were too simple *or* they were
  ones that readers had already seen/done before

In case some of these same issues bother you as you review the exercise routine in this chapter, I would like to take a moment out to dispel a few common misconceptions. The first one is that some people think you have to spend *a lot* of time doing *a lot* of exercises in order to get better–which is simply untrue.

If your exercise program truly targets the *correct* problems with *effective* exercises, then you should not be spending all day doing dozens of exercises. Of course there are exceptions, but they are few.

Another misconception is that simple, uncomplicated exercises are ineffective. Take stretching for example. Pulling one foot up towards your buttock, and holding it there for a mere thirty-seconds, once a day, may appear to some readers to be too simple a maneuver or too short a time frame to ever stretch out tight muscles. But on the contrary, multiple randomized controlled trials have *consistently* pointed out that stretching for a longer period of time, or more times a day, will *not* produce better results.

And finally, the last common misconception deals with not trying an exercise because, "I've done that one before and it didn't help." The interesting thing I've noted, is that when you question someone carefully about what they actually did, you often find that while a person may in fact have been doing an exercise correctly, they have *not* been following proper evidence-based guidelines. Using stretching as an example again, let's say that a person tries a particular stretch that is indeed targeting the correct tight muscle, only they've been holding the stretch for *fifteen-seconds* instead of the proven *thirty-seconds*.

After getting poor results for a period of time, most people will usually abandon the exercise and think, "That stretch didn't work." The truth, however, is that they really were doing a helpful exercise, it's just that they weren't following the correct evidence-based guidelines to make the exercise effective.

The moral? When proceeding with the exercises in this book, make sure that you do them *exactly* as instructed, even if you've tried some of them before or they seem too simple to be effective. Then and only then can you say with certainty that the exercises in this book were really helpful or not.

The Six-Week Program

Up to this point in the book, we've built a good foundation of knowledge for you to be able to treat your own knee arthritis. With that accomplished, it's now time to go over the six-week program I've laid out for you. Here are a few key rules to always keep in mind before you begin …

- always check with your doctor before beginning an exercise program

- the number one rule is "Do no harm." You should not be in a lot of pain while doing these exercises. Some discomfort is okay, but remember that you're working muscles you probably haven't used in a while, at least in this manner.

- stop the exercise if you have any significant increase in knee pain or symptoms. If done correctly, the exercises in this book do not stretch your knee in odd or unsafe positions, nor do they involve any heavy weights– and should be safe for your knee. *However*, it's your knees and your responsibility to stop if you feel like any harm is being done.

At this point, some readers may be wondering, can a home exercise program *really* work? Well, the best way in medicine to prove that something "works" is to conduct what is known as a randomized controlled trial–because this type of study provides the highest proof possible that a treatment is really effective. Here's one such example that involved knee arthritis patients…

- 46 patients with knee pain and X-ray signs of arthritis were randomized to get either a home exercise program, or a nutrition education program (Baker 2001)

- researchers found that those patients who did the home exercise program showed a 71% improvement in quadriceps strength, and a 43% reduction in pain

As this study shows, it's quite possible for knee arthritis patients to drastically increase strength and decrease symptoms all on their own with a simple home exercise program. In fact, some randomized controlled trials have even shown home exercise to work as well as nonsteroidal anti-inflammatory drugs (Doi 2008). Having said that, here's the six-week home exercise program designed to treat your knee arthritis by improving the functioning of your knee…

DO THESE EXERCISES ON MONDAY. WEDNESDAY. and FRIDAY

Increases Knee Flexibility		Increases Knee Strength		Increases Knee Proprioception	Increases Knee Endurance

Knee Stretch #1: Increase Flexion (pick one)

Knee Stretch #2: Increase Extension (pick one)

Quadriceps Strengthening (pick one)

Quadriceps Strengthening (pick one)

Knee Proprioception Exercise

Knee Endurance Exercise (pick one)

hold for 30 sec. x 1
p. 58

hold for 30 sec. x 1
p. 60

hold for 3-5 seconds x 30 reps
p. 44

1 set x 20 reps
p. 47

start with 30 seconds
p. 65

20 to 30 mins.
p. 69

or

or

or

or

or

hold for 30 sec. x 1
p. 59

hold for 30 sec. x 1
p. 61

1 set x 20 reps
p. 45

1 set x 20 reps
p. 48

20 to 30 mins.
p. 70

or

or

1 set x 20 reps
p.46

20 to 30 mins.
p. 71

or

20 to 30 mins.
p. 72

or

20 to 30 mins.
p. 73

DO THESE EXERCISES ON TUESDAY and THURSDAY

Increases Knee Flexibility

⋁   ⋁

Knee Stretch #1:   **Knee Stretch #2:**
Increase Flexion   **Increase Extension**
(pick one)   **(pick one)**

hold for   hold for
30 sec. x 1   30 sec. x 1
p. 58   p. 60

or   or

hold for   hold for
30 sec. x 1   30 sec. x 1
p. 59   p. 61

Track Your Progress!

Since it can be hard to remember from one session to the next what weight you used, or how many seconds you stood on one leg, it's helpful to quickly jot down this information. I've also found that when patients keep track of their exercises, it helps keep them on track too! The following is an example of how to record your progress by using the exercise sheets provided in this book...

Week 3: Exercise Session #3
Wednesday

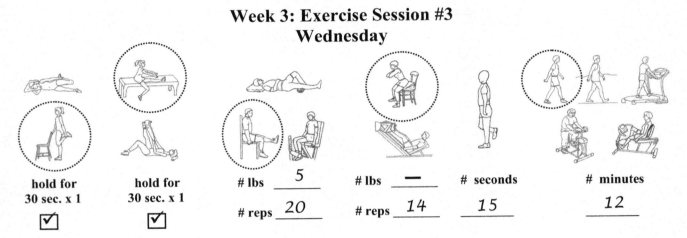

Using the exercise sheets provided is easy. *Starting left to right*, you'll see the two quadriceps stretches, one in sitting and one in standing–pick the one that works the best for you and put a check in the box *after* you do it (feel free to circle the exercise you picked if it helps you remember). Now move to the right, and you'll see the two hamstring stretches–here again, pick one of them and put a check in the box after you do it.

Next, you'll see the *first* group of quadriceps strengthening exercises–pick one of them that suits you best, and put a check in the box after you do it. As you can see in the example, this person used five-pounds on the exercise of their choice, and then did 20 reps. After finishing with that exercise, keep moving to the right and do the same with the *second* group of quadriceps strengthening exercises.

Next up is the proprioception exercise, and as you can see in the example, this person could stand on one leg for 15 seconds–so they simply jotted down a "15" under the picture of that exercise. Next time, maybe they can stand on one leg for 20 or 25 seconds. And lastly, to the far right, are the five endurance exercises–pick one and record how long you did it.

When Do I Stop?

I recommend that you do the full program for six weeks. Studies have shown that this is how long it takes to make good, measurable gains in knee function. If your knee feels great after six weeks, try doing the strengthening, stretching, proprioception, and endurance exercises *once a week* for maintenance–and see how that goes.

On the other hand, if you have good pain relief after doing the program for six weeks, but you're still not quite where you want to be, continue with the program until you either reach your goal, or no further progress is being made. And, if you have not seen a lick of progress after doing the program in the book for three months, then it is not the solution to your knee pain.

The pages that follow contain exercise sheets for six weeks of workouts. Make additional copies as needed–and don't miss the *Quickstart Guide* that is included at the end of this chapter to get you started.

Week 1: Exercise Session #1
Monday

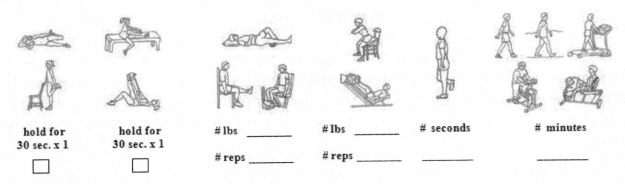

hold for
30 sec. x 1
☐

hold for
30 sec. x 1
☐

lbs _____

reps _____

lbs _____

reps _____

seconds

_____

minutes

_____

Week 1: Exercise Session #2
Tuesday

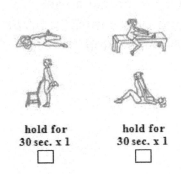

hold for
30 sec. x 1
☐

hold for
30 sec. x 1
☐

Week 1: Exercise Session #3
Wednesday

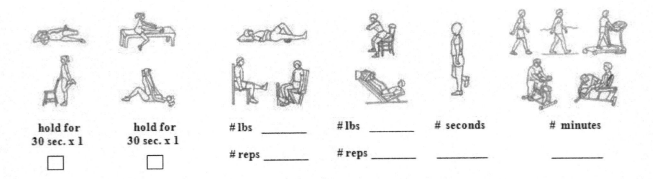

hold for
30 sec. x 1
☐

hold for
30 sec. x 1
☐

lbs _____

reps _____

lbs _____

reps _____

seconds

_____

minutes

_____

Week 1: Exercise Session #4
Thursday

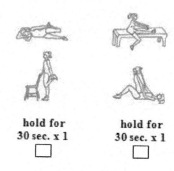

hold for   hold for
30 sec. x 1   30 sec. x 1
☐   ☐

Week 1: Exercise Session #5
Friday

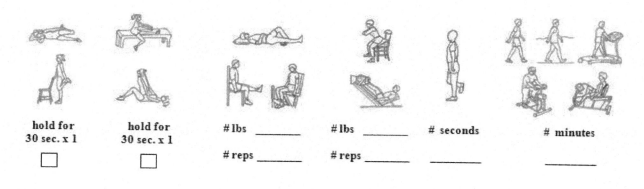

hold for 30 sec. x 1	hold for 30 sec. x 1	# lbs _____ # reps _____	# lbs _____ # reps _____	# seconds _____	# minutes _____
☐	☐				

Week 2: Exercise Session #1
Monday

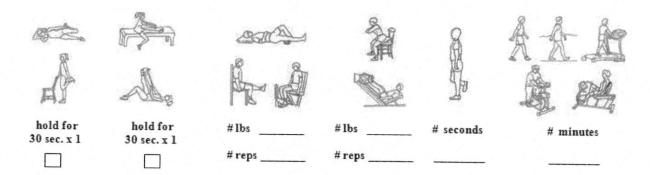

hold for 30 sec. x 1	hold for 30 sec. x 1	# lbs _____ # reps _____	# lbs _____ # reps _____	# seconds _____	# minutes _____
☐	☐				

Week 2: Exercise Session #2
Tuesday

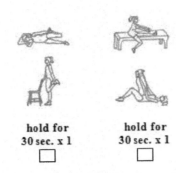

hold for   hold for
30 sec. x 1   30 sec. x 1
☐   ☐

Week 2: Exercise Session #3
Wednesday

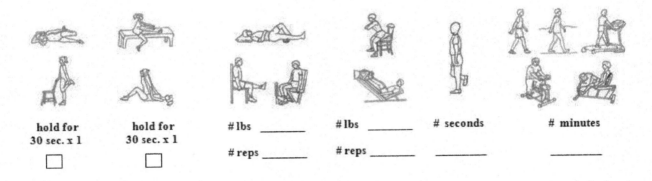

hold for   hold for   # lbs _____   # lbs _____   # seconds   # minutes
30 sec. x 1 30 sec. x 1
☐   ☐   # reps _____   # reps _____   _____   _____

Week 2: Exercise Session #4
Thursday

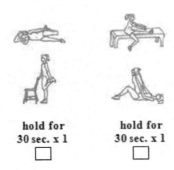

hold for   hold for
30 sec. x 1   30 sec. x 1
☐   ☐

Week 2: Exercise Session #5
Friday

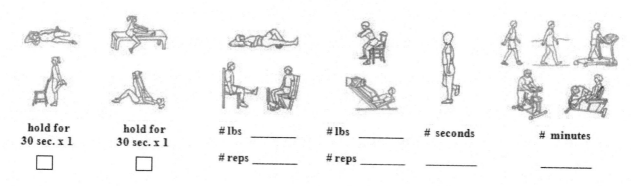

hold for 30 sec. x 1	hold for 30 sec. x 1	# lbs _____ # reps _____	# lbs _____ # reps _____	# seconds _____	# minutes _____
☐	☐				

Week 3: Exercise Session #1
Monday

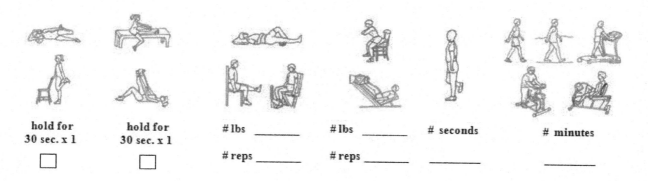

hold for 30 sec. x 1	hold for 30 sec. x 1	# lbs _____ # reps _____	# lbs _____ # reps _____	# seconds _____	# minutes _____
☐	☐				

Week 3: Exercise Session #2
Tuesday

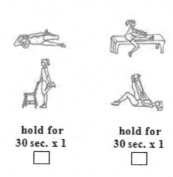

hold for 30 sec. x 1	hold for 30 sec. x 1
☐	☐

Week 3: Exercise Session #3
Wednesday

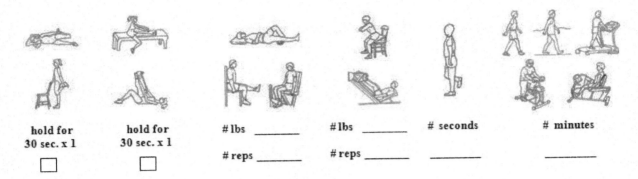

hold for 30 sec. x 1	hold for 30 sec. x 1	# lbs _____ # reps _____	# lbs _____ # reps _____	# seconds _____	# minutes _____
☐	☐				

Week 3: Exercise Session #4
Thursday

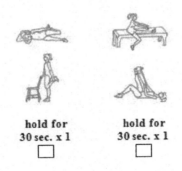

hold for 30 sec. x 1	hold for 30 sec. x 1
☐	☐

Week 3: Exercise Session #5
Friday

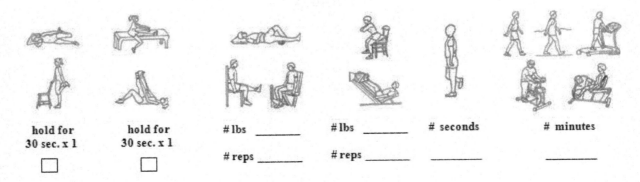

hold for 30 sec. x 1	hold for 30 sec. x 1	# lbs _____ # reps _____	# lbs _____ # reps _____	# seconds _____	# minutes _____
☐	☐				

Week 4: Exercise Session #1
Monday

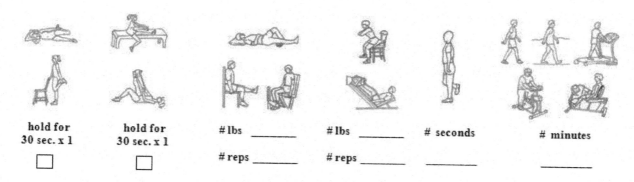

hold for
30 sec. x 1
☐

hold for
30 sec. x 1
☐

lbs _____

reps _____

lbs _____

reps _____

seconds

_____

minutes

_____

Week 4: Exercise Session #2
Tuesday

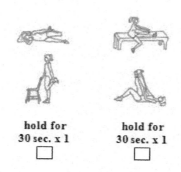

hold for
30 sec. x 1
☐

hold for
30 sec. x 1
☐

Week 4: Exercise Session #3
Wednesday

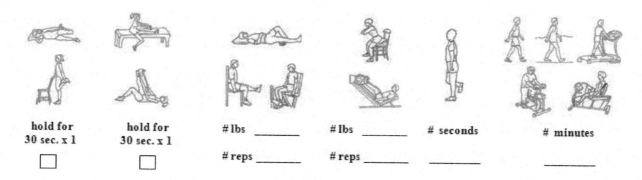

hold for
30 sec. x 1
☐

hold for
30 sec. x 1
☐

lbs _____

reps _____

lbs _____

reps _____

seconds

_____

minutes

_____

Week 4: Exercise Session #4
Thursday

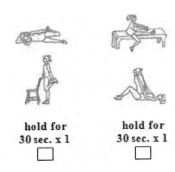

hold for   hold for
30 sec. x 1   30 sec. x 1
☐   ☐

Week 4: Exercise Session #5
Friday

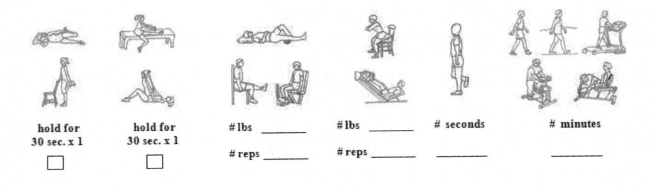

hold for   hold for   # lbs _____   #lbs _____   # seconds   # minutes
30 sec. x 1 30 sec. x 1
☐   ☐   # reps _____   # reps _____ _____   _____

Week 5: Exercise Session #1
Monday

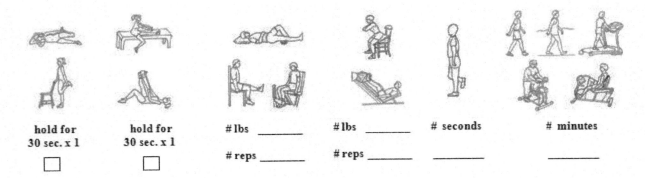

hold for   hold for   # lbs _____   #lbs _____   # seconds   # minutes
30 sec. x 1 30 sec. x 1
☐   ☐   # reps _____   # reps _____ _____   _____

Week 5: Exercise Session #2
Tuesday

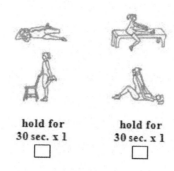

hold for   hold for
30 sec. x 1   30 sec. x 1
☐   ☐

Week 5: Exercise Session #3
Wednesday

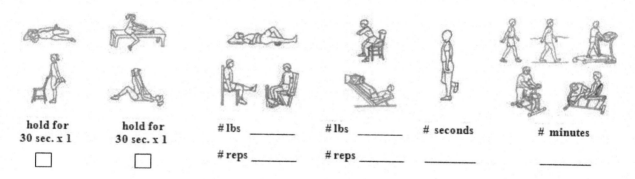

hold for   hold for   # lbs _____   # lbs _____   # seconds   # minutes
30 sec. x 1 30 sec. x 1 # reps _____ # reps _____ _____ _____
☐   ☐

Week 5: Exercise Session #4
Thursday

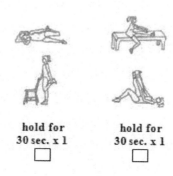

hold for   hold for
30 sec. x 1   30 sec. x 1
☐   ☐

Week 5: Exercise Session #5
Friday

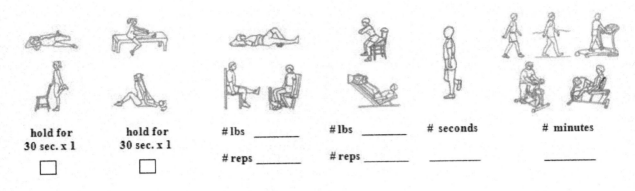

hold for
30 sec. x 1
☐

hold for
30 sec. x 1
☐

#lbs _____

reps _____

#lbs _____

reps _____

seconds

_____

minutes

_____

Week 6: Exercise Session #1
Monday

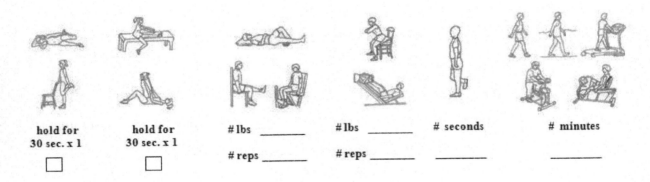

hold for
30 sec. x 1
☐

hold for
30 sec. x 1
☐

#lbs _____

reps _____

#lbs _____

reps _____

seconds

_____

minutes

_____

Week 6: Exercise Session #2
Tuesday

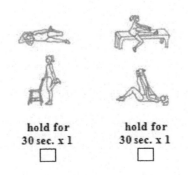

hold for
30 sec. x 1
☐

hold for
30 sec. x 1
☐

Week 6: Exercise Session #3
Wednesday

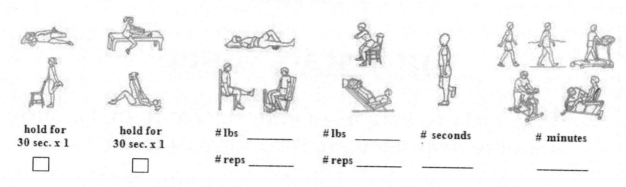

| hold for 30 sec. x 1 | hold for 30 sec. x 1 | # lbs _____ # reps _____ | # lbs _____ # reps _____ | # seconds _____ | # minutes _____ |
| ☐ | ☐ | | | | |

Week 6: Exercise Session #4
Thursday

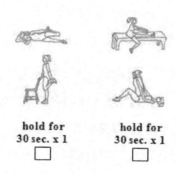

| hold for 30 sec. x 1 | hold for 30 sec. x 1 |
| ☐ | ☐ |

Week 6: Exercise Session #5
Friday

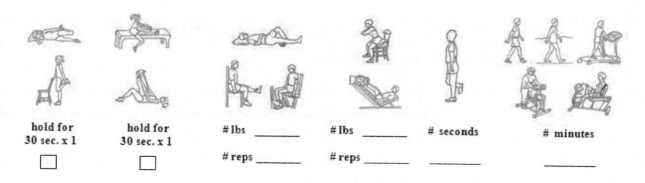

| hold for 30 sec. x 1 | hold for 30 sec. x 1 | # lbs _____ # reps _____ | # lbs _____ # reps _____ | # seconds _____ | # minutes _____ |
| ☐ | ☐ | | | | |

Quickstart Guide

✓ first, get an okay from your doctor to make sure that the exercises are safe for you to do

✓ if you're not using weight machines for the strengthening exercise, purchase a pair of adjustable cuff weights if you don't already have them

✓ take a look at the six-week plan and pick a day of the week to start

✓ on the day you start, it is suggested that you do the exercises in the order pictured, but you don't necessarily *have* to. Use the page numbers provided under each exercise picture on pages 78 and 79 to refer to in case you forgot how to do some of the exercises.

✓ use the handy exercise sheets provided to keep track of your workouts

✓ try to stick with the routine for at least six weeks for best results

Why Measuring Your Progress Is *Very* Important

Okay. You've learned all about knee arthritis, started the exercises, and are on the road to recovery. So now what should you expect?

Well, we all know you should expect to get better. But what exactly does *better* mean? As a physical therapist treating patients, it means two distinct things to me:

- your knee starts to *feel* better

and

- your knee starts to *work* better

And so, when a patient returns for a follow-up visit, I will re-assess them, looking for specific changes in their knee **pain**, as well as their knee **function**.

In this book, I'm going to recommend that readers do the same thing periodically. Why? Simply because people in pain can't always see the progress they're making. For instance, sometimes a person's knee pain doesn't seem to be getting any better, but they can now do some motions or tasks that they couldn't do before–a sure sign that things *are* healing. Or, sometimes a person still has significant knee pain, but they're not looking at the fact that it's actually occurring less frequently–yet another good indication that positive changes are taking place.

Whatever the case may be, if a person isn't looking at the big picture, and doesn't think they're getting any better, they're likely to get discouraged and stop doing their exercises altogether–even though they really might have been on the right track!

On the other hand though, what if you periodically check your progress and are keenly aware that your knee *is* making some changes for the better? What if you can *positively* see *objective* results? My guess is that you're going to be giving yourself a healthy dose of motivation to keep on truckin' with the exercises.

Having said that, I'm going to show you exactly what to check for from time-to-time so that you can monitor the changes that are taking place. I call them "outcomes" and there are two of them.

Outcome #1:
Look for Changes in Your Pain

First of all, you should look for changes in your pain. I know this may sound silly, but sometimes it's my job to get a person to see that their pain *is* actually improving. You see, a lot of people come to physical therapy thinking they're going to be pain-free right away. Then, when they're not instantly better and still having pain, they often start to worry and become discouraged. Truth is, I have yet to put a patient on an exercise program for knee arthritis and have them get instantly better. Better yes, but not *instantly* better.

Over the years, I have found that patients usually respond to the exercises in a quite predictable pattern. One of three things will almost always occur as patients begin to turn the corner and get better:

- your knee pain will be just as intense as always,
  however now it is occurring much less frequently

  or

- your knee pain is now *less* intense, even though
  it is still occurring just as frequently

  or

- you start to notice less intense knee pain *and* it is
  now occurring less frequently

The point here is to make sure that you keep a sharp eye out for any of these three changes as you progress with the exercises. If *any* of them occur, it will be a sure sign that the exercises are helping and you're on the right track. You can then look forward to the pain gradually getting better, usually over the weeks to come.

Outcome #2:
Look for Changes in Knee Function

Looking at how well your knee works is very important because many times knee function improves *before* the pain does. For example, sometimes a patient will do the exercises for a while, and although their knee will still hurt a lot, they are able to do many things that they hadn't been able to in a while–a really good indicator that healing is taking place *and* that the pain should be easing up soon.

While measuring your knee function may sound like a pain in the butt, it doesn't have to be. In this book, I'm recommending that readers use a quick and easy assessment tool known as *The Knee Injury and Osteoarthritis Outcome Score-Physical Function Short-Form* (Perruccio 2008). Well, let's just call it the KOOS-PS for short.

While the name certainly sounds like a nightmare, the KOOS-PS is a really useful tool you can use to keep track of how your knee is *functioning*. Studies show that it is a valid test (Davis 2009), has good test-retest reliability (Ornetti 2009, Goncalves 2010), and is responsive to clinical changes (Davis 2009). And best of all, *it takes only a couple of minutes to complete*. Now that's my kinda test!

So what exactly does taking the KOOS-PS involve? Not much.

- you read the instructions and then simply check the degree of difficulty you have doing each of the seven activities

- next, you add up your points and use a table to get your score

On the next page is the KOOS-PS, let's have a look....

KOOS-Physical Function Shortform (KOOS-PS)

INSTRUCTIONS: This survey asks for your view about your knee. This information will help us keep track of how well you are able to perform different activities.

Answer every question by checking the appropriate box, only one box for each question. If you are unsure about how to answer a question, please give the best answer you can so that you answer all the questions.

The following questions concern your level of function in performing usual daily activities and higher level activities. For each of the following activities, please indicate the degree of difficulty you have experienced in the **last week** due to your knee problem.

1. Rising from bed

None	Mild	Moderate	Severe	Extreme
❑	❑	❑	❑	❑

2. Putting on socks/stockings

None	Mild	Moderate	Severe	Extreme
❑	❑	❑	❑	❑

3. Rising from sitting

None	Mild	Moderate	Severe	Extreme
❑	❑	❑	❑	❑

4. Bending to floor

None	Mild	Moderate	Severe	Extreme
❑	❑	❑	❑	❑

5. Twisting/pivoting on your injured knee

None	Mild	Moderate	Severe	Extreme
❑	❑	❑	❑	❑

6. Kneeling

None	Mild	Moderate	Severe	Extreme
❑	❑	❑	❑	❑

7. Squatting

None	Mild	Moderate	Severe	Extreme
❑	❑	❑	❑	❑

your total points	your score
0	0
1	5.6
2	10.5
3	14.8
4	18.63
5	22
6	24.9
7	27.5
8	29.7
9	31.8
10	33.6
11	35.3
12	37
13	38.6
14	40.3
15	42
16	44
17	46.1
18	48.5
19	51.2
20	54.4
21	57.9
22	62
23	66.6
24	71.8
25	77.7
26	84.3
27	91.8
28	100

After you're done completing the KOOS-PS, you're going to give yourself points based on the boxes you've just checked. So…

- give yourself 1 point every time you checked "mild"
- give yourself 2 points every time you checked "moderate"
- give yourself 3 points every time you checked "severe"
- give yourself 4 points every time you checked "extreme"

Go ahead and add up the points, which will equal a number anywhere from 0 to 28.

Now, using the table on the right, take your point total number, and find it in the *left* hand column. Found it? Okay, your score will be the number that is directly to the *right* of it, in the right hand column.

For example, let's say you added up the points and your total points equaled 16. Just find the number 16 in the left hand column, and your score will be just to the right, which would be 44.

So what was your score? Keep in mind that scores will range anywhere from a 0 to a 100. Higher scores mean you're in bad shape, so your goal is to score as *low* as possible. In other words, a score of 0 means you're having *no* difficulty doing any of the activities listed in the survey, while a score of 100 means you're having a lot of trouble.

If you did score high though, don't worry. Just keep taking the KOOS-PS every few weeks, and as you progress with the exercises, you should see your score go lower and lower as time passes. Remember, sometimes knee function gets better *before* the pain does.

Quick Review

✓ being aware of your progress is an important part of treating your knee arthritis–it motivates you to keep doing the exercises.

✓ look for the pain to become less *intense*, less *frequent,* or both to let you know that the exercises are helping

✓ sometimes your knee starts to work better *before* it starts to feel better. Taking the *KOOS-PS* from time-to-time makes you aware of improving knee function.

Comprehensive List of Supporting References

Well, we've come a long way since page one. Now that we're coming to the end, I'd like to take a few minutes to show you all the research that went into this book.

The following is a list of all the randomized controlled trials and scientific studies that have been published in peer-reviewed journals that this book is based on. To make a long story short, there's no nonsense going on here–*every* piece of information you've just read has a good evidence-based reason for being here!

Having said that, I've included this handy reference section so that readers can check out the information for themselves if they wish. Good luck!

Chapter 1

Bhattacharyya T, et al. The clinical importance of meniscal tears demonstrated by magnetic resonance imaging in osteoarthritis of the knee. *Journal of Bone and Joint Surgery* 2007;85-A:4-9.

Chakravarty E, et al. Long distance running and knee osteoarthritis. A prospective study. *Am J Prev Med* 2008;35:133-138.

Felson D, et al. The association of bone marrow lesions with pain in knee osteoarthritis. *Ann Int Med* 2001;134:541-549.

Hannan M, et al. Analysis of the discordance between radiographic changes and knee pain in osteoarthritis of the knee. *J Rheumatology* 2000;27:1513-1517.

Lane N, et al. The relationship of running to osteoarthritis of the knee and hip and bone mineral density of the lumbar spine: a 9-year longitudinal study. *J Rheumatology* 1998;25:334-41.

Miller M, et al. Modifiers of change in physical functioning in older adults with knee pain: the observational arthritis study in seniors (OASIS). *Arthritis Care and Research* 2001;45:331-339.

Panush, R, et al. Is running associated with osteoarthritis? An eight-year follow-up study. *J of Clin Rheum* 1995;1:35-39.

Messier S, et al. Risk factors and mechanisms of knee injury in runners. *Medicine and Science in Sports and Exercise* 2008;40:1873-1879.

Slemenda C, et al. Quadriceps weakness and osteoarthritis of the knee. *Ann Int Med* 1997;127;97-104.

Chapter 2

Barker K, et al. Association between radiographic joint space narrowing, function, pain, and muscle power in severe osteoarthritis of the knee. *Clin Rehabil* 2004;18:793-800.

Bedson J, et al. The discordance between clinical and radiographic knee osteoarthritis: a systematic search and summary of the literature. *BMC Musculoskeletal Disorders* 2008;9:116.

Dieppe P, et al. The Bristol 'OA500 study': progression and impact of the disease after 8 years. Osteoarthritis and Cartilage 2000;8:63-68.

Hannan M, et al. Analysis of the discordance between radiographic changes and knee pain in osteoarthritis of the knee. *J Rheumatology* 2000;27:1513-1517.

Massardo L, et al. Osteoarthritis of the knee joint: an eight-year prospective study. *Ann of the Rheum Dis* 1989;48:893-897.

Spector T, et al. Radiological progression of osteoarthritis: an 11-year follow-up study of the knee. *Ann Rheum Dis* 1992;51:1107-10.

Chapter 3

Berger R, et. al. Effect of various repetitive rates in weight training on improvements in strength and endurance. *J Assoc Phys Mental Rehabil* 1966;20:205-207.

Braith R, et. al. Comparison of 2 vs 3 days/week of variable resistance training during 10- and 18- week programs. *Int J Sports Med* 1989;10:450-454.

Carolan B, Cafarelli E. Adaptations in coactivation after isometric resistance training. *J Appl Physiol* 1992;73:911-917.

Carroll T, et. al. Resistance training frequency: strength and myosin heavy chain responses to two and three bouts per week. *Eur J Appl Physiol* 1998;78:270-275.

DeMichele P, et. al. Isometric torso rotation strength: effect of training frequency on its development. *Arch Phys Med Rehabil* 1997;78:64-69.

Esquivel A, et al. High and low volume resistance training and vascular function. *Int J of Sports Med* 2007;28:217-221.

Garfinkel S, Cafarelli E. Relative changes in maximal force, EMG, and muscle cross-sectional area after isometric training. *Medicine and Science in Sports and Exercise* 1992;24:1220-1227.

Hall K, et al. Differential strength decline in patients with osteoarthritis of the knee: revision of a hypothesis. *Arthritis Care and Research* 1993;6:89-96.

Hass C, et. al. Single versus multiple sets in long-term recreational weightlifters. *Medicine and Science in Sports and Exercise* 2000;32:235-242.

Hassan B, et al. Static postural sway, proprioception, and maximal voluntary quadriceps contraction in patients with knee osteoarthritis and normal control subjects. *Ann Rheum Dis* 2001;60:612-618.

Hurley M, et al. The influence of arthrogenous muscle inhibition on quadriceps rehabilitation of patients with early, unilateral osteoarthritic knees. *Br J Rheum* 1993;32:127-31.

Hurley M, et al. Sensorimotor changes and functional performance in patients with knee osteoarthritis. Ann Rheum Dis 1997;56:641-648.

Fisher N, et al. Reduced muscle function in patients with osteoarthritis. *Scan J Rehab Med* 1997;29:213-221.

O'Shea P. Effects of selected weight training programs on the development of strength and muscle hypertrophy. *Research Quarterly* 1966;37:95-102.

Palmieri G. Weight training and repetition speed. *Journal of Applied Sport Science Research* 1987;1:36-38.

Reid C, et. al. Weight training and strength, cardiorespiratory functioning and body composition of men. *Br J Sports Med* 1987;21:40-44.

Slemenda C, et al. Quadriceps weakness and osteoarthritis of the knee. *Ann Int Med* 1997;127;97-104.

Starkey D, et. al. Effect of resistance training volume on strength and muscle thickness. *Medicine and Science in Sports and Exercise* 1996;28:1311-1320.

Stowers T, et. al. The short-term effects of three different strength-power training methods. *Natl Strength Cond J* 1983;5:24-27.

Silvester L, et. al. The effect of variable resistance and free-weight training programs on strength and vertical jump. *Natl Strength Cond J* 1982;3:30-33.

Young W, Bilby G. The effect of voluntary effort to influence speed of contraction on strength, muscular power, and hypertrophy development. *J of Strength and Conditioning Research* 1993;7:172-178.

Chapter 4

Bandy W, et. al. The effect of static stretch and dynamic range of motion training on the flexibility of the hamstring muscles. *Journal of Orthopaedic and Sports Physical Therapy* 1998;27:295-300.

Bandy W, et. al. The effect of time and frequency of static stretching on flexibility of the hamstring muscles. *Physical Therapy* 1997;77:1090-1096.

Bandy W, Irion J. The effect of time on static stretch on the flexibility of the hamstring muscles. *Physical Therapy* 1994;74:845-852.

Liikavainio T, et al. Physical function and properties of quadriceps femoris muscle in men with knee osteoarthritis. *Arch Phys Med Rehabil* 2008;89:2185-94.

Messier S, et al. Osteoarthritis of the knee: effects on gait, strength, and flexibility. *Arch Phys Med Rehabil* 1992;73: 29-36.

Chapter 5

Hassan B, et al. Static postural sway, proprioception, and maximal voluntary quadriceps contraction in patients with knee osteoarthritis and normal control subjects. *Ann Rheum Dis* 2001;60:612-618.

Hurley M, et al. Improvements in quadriceps sensorimotor function and disability of patients with knee osteoarthritis following a clinically practicable exercise regime. *Br J of Rheum* 1998;37:1181-1187.

Jan M, et al. Effects of weight-bearing vs nonweight bearing exercise on function, walking speed, and position sense in participants with knee osteoarthritis: a randomized controlled trial. *Arch Phys Med Rehabil* 2009;90:897-904.

Koralewicz L, et al. Comparison of proprioception in arthritic and age-matched normal knees. *Journal of Bone and Joint Surgery* 2000;82-A:1582-1588.

Tsauo J, et al. The effects of sensorimotor training on knee proprioception and function for patients with knee osteoarthritis: a preliminary report. *Clin Rehab* 2008;22:448-457.

Chapter 6

Fisher N, et al. Reduced muscle function in patients with osteoarthritis. *Scan J Rehab Med* 1997;29:213-221.

Kovar P, et al.. Supervised fitness walking in patients with osteoarthritis of the knee. A randomized, controlled trial. *Ann Int Med* 1992;116:529-534.

Philbin E, et al. Cardiovascular fitness and health in patients with end-stage osteoarthritis. *Arthritis and Rheumatism* 1995;38:799-805.

Talbot L, et al. A home-based pedometer-driven walking program to increase physical activity in older adults with osteoarthritis of the knee: a preliminary study. *J Am Geriatr Soc* 2003;51:387-392.

Chapter 7

Baker K, et al. The efficacy of home based progressive strength training in older adults with knee osteoarthritis: a randomized controlled trial. *J Rheum* 2001;28:1655-65.

Doi T, et al. Effect of home exercise of quadriceps on knee osteoarthritis compared with nonsteroidal antiinflammatory drugs. A randomized controlled trial. *Am J Phys Med Rehabil* 2008;87:258-269.

<u>Chapter 8</u>

Davis A, et al. Comparative, validity and responsiveness of the HOOS-PS and KOOS-PS to the WOMAC physical function subscale in total joint replacement for osteoarthritis. *Osteoarthritis and Cartilage* 2009;17:843-847.

Goncalves R, et al. Reliability, validity and responsiveness of the Portuguese version of the knee injury and osteoarthritis outcome score-physical function short-form (KOOS-PS). Osteoarthritis and Cartilage 2010;18:372-376.

Ornetti P, et al. Psychometric properties of the French translation of the reduced KOOS and HOOS (KOOS-PS and HOOS-PS) *Osteoarthritis and Cartilage* 2009;17:1604-1608.

Perruccio A, et al. The development of a short measure of physical function for knee OA KOOS-Physical function shortform (KOOS-PS)- an OARSI/OMERACT initiative. *Osteoarthritis and Cartilage* 2008;16:542-550.

CPSIA information can be obtained at www.ICGtesting.com
Printed in the USA
BVOW09s0542170116

433159BV00002BB/30/P